A Practitioner's Guide to
Clinical Cupping

A Practitioner's Guide to
Clinical Cupping

Effective Techniques for Pain
Management and Injury

DANIEL LAWRENCE

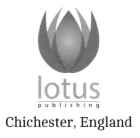

lotus
publishing
Chichester, England

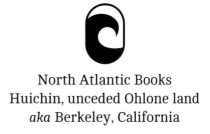

North Atlantic Books
Huichin, unceded Ohlone land
aka Berkeley, California

First published in 2023 by
Lotus Publishing
Apple Tree Cottage, Inlands Road, Nutbourne, Chichester, PO18 8RJ, and
North Atlantic Books
Huichin, unceded Ohlone land
aka Berkeley, California

Illustrations Amanda Williams
Photographs and Videos Richard Draisey @refreshstagnes
Models Rose Buckmaster, Kimberley Lawrence, Richard Draisey, Daniel Lawrence
Text Design Medlar Publishing Solutions Pvt Ltd., India
Cover Design Jasmine Hromjak
Printed and Bound in India by Replika Press Pvt Ltd

A Practitioner's Guide to Clinical Cupping: Effective Techniques for Pain Management and Injury is sponsored and published by North Atlantic Books, an educational non-profit based on the unceded Ohlone land Huichin (*aka* Berkeley, CA), that collaborates with partners to develop cross-cultural perspectives, nurture holistic views of art, science, the humanities, and healing, and seed personal and global transformation by publishing work on the relationship of body, spirit, and nature.

North Atlantic Books' publications are distributed to the US trade and internationally by Penguin Random House Publishers Services. For further information, visit our website at www.northatlanticbooks.com.

MEDICAL DISCLAIMER: The following information is intended for general information purposes only. Individuals should always see their health care provider before administering any suggestions made in this book. Any application of the material set forth in the following pages is at the reader's discretion and is their sole responsibility.

British Library Cataloging-in-Publication Data
A CIP record for this book is available from the British Library
ISBN 978 1 913088 33 0 (Lotus Publishing)
ISBN 978 1 62317 839 0 (North Atlantic Books)

Library of Congress Cataloging-in-Publication Data
Names: Lawrence, Daniel (Physical therapist), author.
Title: A practitioner's guide to clinical cupping : effective techniques for pain management and injury / Daniel Lawrence.
Description: Chichester : Lotus Publishing ; Berkeley, California : North Atlantic Books, [2023] | Includes bibliographical references and index. | Summary: "A Practitioner's Guide to Clinical Cupping presents a new approach to cupping therapy that offers enhanced treatment outcomes and methods more readily accepted by western medicine and modern manual therapy bodyworkers"--Provided by publisher.
Identifiers: LCCN 2022027563 (print) | LCCN 2022027564 (ebook) | ISBN 9781623178390 (trade paperback) | ISBN 9781623178406 (ebook)
Subjects: MESH: Cupping Therapy--methods | Pain Management--methods
Classification: LCC RM184 (print) | LCC RM184 (ebook) | NLM WB 371 | DDC 615.8/9--dc23/eng/20220727
LC record available at https://lccn.loc.gov/2022027563
LC ebook record available at https://lccn.loc.gov/2022027564

Contents

Foreword

I feel the classic prompt for anyone asked to write a foreword is to diminish one's influence on the author of the book. Well, I'm not going to do that. Daniel and I have known each other for close to a decade and I quickly recognized that he was someone that was authentically committed to helping others move in a meaningful way. Thankfully, he is also a brilliant mind that has the keen ability to deliver science informed information in a consumable manner. Selfishly, knowing that I could never articulate my view of pain and movement as eloquently as him, I decided to infiltrate his mind to act as a vehicle of ideas I had on these topics. As I expected, Daniel accomplished the task with little need for my input, mind you, in such a concise and practical manner that I am honored to be able to provide this foreword for my friend as a gesture of my gratitude.

You may be asking how could anyone really provide more insight on an ancient manual therapy like cupping? Well, Daniel in his attempt to create a meaningful therapeutic experience has done just that. Let me explain.

Many, scientifically validated, therapeutic interventions provide inconsistent outcomes. In my 20 years of experience in this field, I've noticed that many therapists have forgotten that we are interacting with a human being attached to the tissues we are treating. Well, Daniel has not forgotten this fact and beautifully reframed the application of an ancient approach of cupping therapy by providing a science-based methodology that integrates the person into the intervention that fosters a more substantial therapeutic alliance.

Throughout this book, he layers practical applications on how to include the client as an active participant in the cupping therapy which has been shown to augment the therapeutic outcome. The combination of the science and art of this manual therapy will provide you with a vast resource of options to best match the needs of the client to be able to achieve the mutual goal.

I am excited for you, the reader, to gain the same benefit that I've been fortunate enough to experience as a bystander to the bright light associated with this phenomenal healer.

Dr. Steven Capobianco
D.C, MA, DACRB, CSCS

Introduction

Cupping—An Ancient Treatment, a New Way

As a British physical therapist, I completed my training during the beginning of the new wave of evidence-based practitioners. My fellow students and I witnessed many of the profession's traditions and practices decline in usage and popularity at the hands of scientific researchers. This led to a new age of physiotherapy whose practitioners sought to help their patients using methods based on scientific "evidence." It is difficult to disagree with this approach when the population's health-care demands seem infinite and access to health care seems increasingly finite. As a result, time with patients is precious and needs to stand the best chance of being effective.

As a consequence of the evidence-based movement, many traditional and time-tested treatments were sidelined, forgotten, or just no longer taught. As an example, massage—considered a foundation of traditional physiotherapy—was virtually excluded from many UK training schools.

It seems that the separation of some of these traditional skills from modern practice has forced a polarization between modern medical practices and more traditional treatments, which are now commonly labelled as "complementary medicine." Complementary medicine practice is often taught via passed-on knowledge of tradition and folklore, and often retains many elements of historical practice. Often shielded from the rigors of modern scientific method, complementary therapies—like cupping—lack the opportunity for modernization and the chance to reconceptualize their use.

However, there has been an emergence of modern research in support of the use of cupping therapy for musculoskeletal problems. This is a case of the science following practice, rather than clinicians following the science. It is evident, despite the paucity of research, that cupping has risen in popularity within professional sport, visually evidenced by many of the swimmers in the Rio and Tokyo Olympics displaying the circular markings associated with cupping.

It has been exciting to be a part of the cupping revival. During the memorable years of 2020 and 2021, the cupping (RockPods™) course became my most popular, as many professionals sought to extend their practice to offer this unique treatment.

Cupping—the creation of a vacuum for medicinal practice—is mentioned in the earliest historical medical texts we have and are known to many cultures around the world. Historically and to the present day there remains a range of cupping application styles, from the cutting of the skin and drawing out of blood that is "wet cupping" to the use of a flame dipped inside a glass cup to create a vacuum, known as "fire cupping." The term "cupping" can refer to very different methods of application, which can create confusion or misrepresentation when advertising a cupping service.

This book focuses on the safe and highly effective dry-cupping method and includes a description of fire cupping within this. There are a variety of explanations given for cupping therapy, and historical accounts and different cultures present various theories or stories to explain how cupping works, from energy flow (*qi*)

to the expulsion of evil spirits. There are plenty of interesting theories to be found in historical texts, although the mechanisms often remain unchallenged by scientific methods. This book provides a modern scientific view, including a mention of some credible scientific experiments that help explain what cupping therapy does. This provides an opportunity to uncover the truth and dispel some of the myths associated with this historic treatment method.

The book is divided into twelve chapters, beginning with a brief but respectful nod to the history of cupping practice and theory. We then use research and modern theory to build an up-to-date knowledge of cupping mechanisms. Prior to the presentation of regional body techniques in chapters 6–12, chapter 2, on application principles, outlines the fundamentals of safe and effective cupping, and chapters 3–5 discuss the mechanics and physiology. I am excited to provide a novel and contemporary approach to cupping, which I hope you will find helpful in your practice, and I look forward to hearing your feedback.

This book is different because, as a modern evidence-based practitioner, I have adopted cupping into my practice, leaving behind the more traditional and dogmatic practices while including the proven therapeutic elements and creating new application styles that offer more robust outcomes.

I feel passionate about the benefits and potential of cupping therapy in modern times and more specifically within the framework of a more-contemporary approach to manual therapy and pain management. I hope this book leads you to share that passion, while supplying guidance on the safe and effective use of dry cupping.

Enjoy!
Daniel

1 The History of Cupping Therapy

Exploring the Origins of an Ancient Treatment Practice

Early History

Cupping is mentioned in historical texts from around the world, including Egypt, China, Europe, and America. Throughout history it has been closely associated with Egyptian, Greek, Chinese, and Arabic cultures, among others. It is also embedded in Sunni Islamic texts.

From Egypt, the Ebers Papyrus (circa 1550 BCE) is one of the oldest surviving medical texts and the oldest surviving evidence of cupping. It is commonly agreed, however, that cupping may have already been practiced by civilizations for thousands of years before this, and we cannot assume that the ancient Egyptians invented it. In fact, while the earliest documentary evidence of many ancient medical practices comes from ancient Egypt, this may be the result of the ancient Egyptians' culture of recording and documenting, using materials that withstand aging

and decay. And the Ebers Papyrus itself is thought to have been copied from earlier texts (see box).

The ancient Greeks are thought to be one of the first cultures to have contact with the ancient Egyptians, and it is believed that Greek medicine was significantly influenced by Egyptian practices. The Greek physician Hippocrates (460–375 BCE) (figure 1.2)—often described as the father of medicine—used cupping extensively, writing about and teaching his students how to perform cupping therapy.

Another noteworthy physician who advocated the use of cupping was Galen (129–216 CE) (figure 1.3), an early medical "influencer" who posthumously had a far-reaching impact on medicine and philosophy throughout Europe and the Middle East until the mid-seventeenth century.

The Ebers Papyrus

The Ebers Papyrus (figure 1.1) is part of a collection of six ancient Egyptian medical texts from around 1500 to 2000 BCE. It is thought that these texts may have been based on earlier texts from around 3000 BCE (Frey 1986). The Ebers Papyrus was said to have been found between the legs of a mummy in the Assasif district of the Theban Necropolis next to the Nile in Egypt. A necropolis is a cemetery, usually with impressive architectural monuments. The word "necropolis" is derived from ancient Greek and translates as "city of the dead"—which sounds like a rather terrifying place to visit, but probably interesting for sightseers and historians.

Following its discovery in the mid-nineteenth century, the papyrus was bought by George Ebers in 1872 and is currently kept at the library of the University of Leipzig in Germany, where a full-sized replica is displayed. When it was found, the papyrus was a continuous scroll nearly 19 meters long. To facilitate its conservation, on arrival in Leipzig it was cut into 29 pieces and preserved under glass.

The papyrus is said to cover more than 800 symptoms and treatments, which include a blend of folklore and science. The prescribed remedies take the form of ointments, enemas, and medicinal substances to be used in a variety of ways, including gargling, smoking, and swallowing. The papyrus contains chapters on contraception, diagnosis of pregnancy and other gynecological matters, intestinal diseases and parasites, eye and skin problems, dentistry and the surgical treatment of abscesses and tumors, bonesetting, and burns.

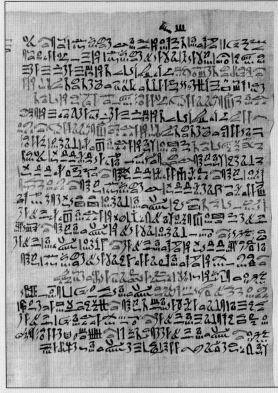

Figure 1.1. The Ebers Papyrus
Image © Archives Charmet/Bridgeman Images

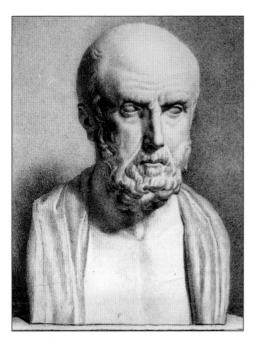

Figure 1.2. Hippocrates
Image © Archives Charmet/Bridgeman Images

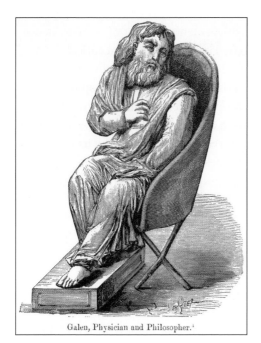

Galen, Physician and Philosopher.

Figure 1.3. Galen
Image © Archives Charmet/Bridgeman Images

Origins in Different Cultures

In the Arab and Muslim world, al-hijamah (wet cupping) is an entrenched religious procedure supported by many hadiths (authenticated sayings) of the Prophet Muhammad (PBUH), who recommended its use for medical conditions more than 1400 years ago (Qureshi et al. 2017).

Many believe that cupping therapy may have first been used in China as an integral part of traditional Chinese medicine. The earliest record of cupping in China is in the Mawangdui Silk Texts (circa 175 BCE) (figure 1.4), which were discovered in a tomb in Hunan, China, in 1973.

There are also many references to cupping therapy in one of the oldest Chinese medical books, *Huang Di Neijing*—"The Yellow Emperor's Classic of Medicine" (said to have been written around 2600 BCE, but possibly dating more recently to around 300 BCE). Recent translations of this book continue to sell in large numbers around the world as people seek to learn from a past that, some might claim, Western medicine has left behind, somewhat to its detriment.

In Europe, it was not just in Greece that cupping was in widespread use by both medical professionals and lay people within their own homes. In Germany, Poland, and the United Kingdom, cupping has been mentioned

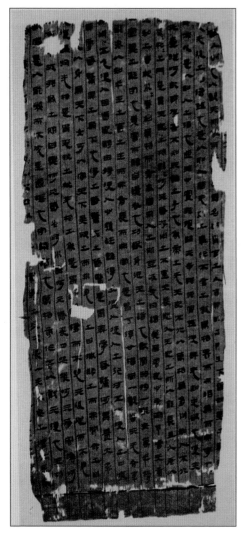

Figure 1.4. The Mawangdui Silk Texts
Image © Wikipedia

as a therapeutic or medical practice throughout history.

In the United States, cupping is known to have been used by the Native Americans and by the medical doctors of the settlers, who were most likely trained in Europe. Both the Native Americans and the European settlers would most likely have used wet cupping for bloodletting. Although their mechanistic theories may have been different, they were probably doing the same thing and getting the same results. Throughout history, cupping therapists have been divided in their opinions on the efficacy of wet cupping, often referred to as bloodletting. This continues to be the case, and in a Western medical setting wet cupping is unlikely to find acceptance among evidence-based practitioners.

More-Recent History

After a long and successful medical reign, cupping therapy fell out of favor from the mid-eighteenth century as the developing field of modern medicine discredited its historical and anecdotal achievements in favor of more evidence-based and often pharmaceutical methods. However, cupping never vanished entirely, and its popularity among modern manual therapists has risen at an astonishing rate over the past few years, fueled in part by its use by athletes and celebrities, as evidenced by the unique circular marks sometimes to be seen on their bodies.

Conclusion

The history of cupping teaches us about the numerous ancient origins of this fascinating treatment tool. It is all too common to view medical history with a sense of superiority, as we compare modern knowledge and practices to those of our less-informed ancestors. However, if we look back further, perhaps thousands rather than hundreds of years, we find knowledge that may have been left behind to the detriment of modern medicine.

For example, ancient Chinese medicine refers many times to balance and harmony within the individual and with the environment. Separately, the Greek physician Galen referred to a medical philosophy of four humors, which—while we may be quick to discredit it on one level of analysis—again presents the concept of health requiring that systems be in balance. Over the past decade we have seen science steer Western medicine away from its linear, biomedical focus on structure toward a more holistic, whole-person, biopsychosocial approach. It is possible that we are rediscovering something our ancestors already implicitly understood.

If cupping is to become and remain a popular and credible treatment in the West, it will need to be taught and utilized in ways that fit the modern approach to manual therapy—thus adding a new chapter to the history of cupping therapy.

References

Frey, E. F. 1986. The earliest medical texts. In *Clio Medica: Acta Academiae Internationalis Historiae Medicinae*, vol. 20, edited by A. M. Luyendijk-Elshout, pp. 79–90. Amsterdam: Rodopi, Brill.

Jouanna, J., and N. Allies. 2012. Egyptian medicine and Greek medicine. In *Greek Medicine from Hippocrates to Galen: Selected Papers*, edited by P. Van der Eijk, pp. 3–20. Leiden: Brill. Retrieved 5 April 2021 from http://www.jstor.org/stable/10.1163/j.cttlw76vxr.6.

Qureshi, N. A., G. I. Ali, T. S. Abushanab, A. T. El-Olemy, M. S. Alqaed, I. S. El-Subai, and A. M. Al-Bedah. 2017. "History of cupping (Hijama): A narrative review of literature." *Journal of Integrative Medicine* 15(3): 172–81.

Wagner, B. B. 2019. "The Ebers Papyrus: Medico-magical beliefs and treatments revealed in ancient Egyptian medical text." *Ancient Origins* [website], last updated 22 July 2019. https://www.ancient-origins.net/artifacts-ancient-writings/ebers-papyrus-0012333.

Cupping Application Principles

The Important Principles to Follow when Cupping

Introduction

In this chapter I will explain the general principles that should be used for the various applications throughout this book. It is important to get the basics correct before moving on to more advanced and tailored treatment approaches. This will avoid unnecessary discomfort for your patient and increase the chances of therapeutic success.

It will become apparent as you read this book that the way I teach and use cupping differs from more traditional practice. These differences are detailed within this chapter and include various fundamentals, such as a short duration of application, minimizing the vacuum pressure, and using fewer cups during the treatment sessions. I learnt much of this from my teaching work with RockTape, and I remain grateful to Doctor Steven Capobianco from the United States for his teachings and inspiration.

Contraindications

Dry cupping is considered a safe treatment modality that can be used in conjunction with many other massage and manual therapy interventions. Cupping does, however, cause a degree of physical stress to the skin and underlying circulatory network, and therefore, the following contraindications should be considered.

- Do not use cups over varicose veins.
- Never use cups over large exposed blood vessels.
- Avoid using cups if a deep vein thrombosis (DVT) is suspected.
- Do not use cups with patients on anticoagulant therapy (blood thinners).
- Never use cups on patients with blood-clotting disorders (e.g. hemophilia).
- Do not use cups on damaged or irritated skin.

- Never use cups on immature scar tissue.
- Avoid using cups over bruises or previous cupping marks.
- Do not cup in or over orifices like the belly button, armpits, or inner groin.
- Never cup over the eyes, mouth, nose, or ears.
- Stop using cups if they cause or increase pain.
- Never cup over or near a fracture site.

The contraindications mentioned above aim to help the new practitioner avoid any obvious mistakes. For many of my students, they are already familiar with these standard contraindications and may have more specific usage concerns regarding cupping for special populations or specific medical conditions.

The overarching advice that I offer to practitioners is that if they are already trained and competent to work with specific groups or particular medical conditions, then they can safely adapt the principles of cupping to suit their patients. For example, cupping could be used for pain relief in an oncology setting, but only by practitioners who are competent to work in this field, with a specialist knowledge of their patient group's medical conditions. A specialist knowledge of cupping alone would not provide the required competency.

Precautionary Usage

When using the cups with special populations and specific medical conditions, it is advisable to first obtain written consent from the patient's medical consultant or general practitioner and to then trial the use of cupping with minimal vacuum and a short (30-second) application time. Feedback from the patient during this trial is also very important. Cupping should not be a painful experience.

Areas to Avoid

I would advise against cupping in the following areas, mostly for comfort reasons but also because such applications offer little to no therapeutic benefit.

Lateral and Anterior Neck

The skin is thin and highly elastic around the lateral and anterior neck. This causes an excess of skin to be drawn up into the cup and an increased rate of ecchymosis. The treatment feels less targeted and is often not very therapeutic. Cupping directly over the carotid artery is also contraindicated.

Anterior Elbow

The thinner skin and more superficial vessels and nerves in this region make the use of cupping with any significant vacuum unadvisable. There is nothing to achieve from cupping this area and I would suggest avoiding it.

Posterior Knee

The thinner skin in this popliteal area makes cupping typically uncomfortable. I would advise against cupping in this region.

Side of the Head

I do not teach or recommend the use of cups over the temporal regions on the side of the head.

Getting Started

Which Cups to Use

There is a wide range of cups and vacuum tools to choose from. Most of them are inexpensive and can be purchased from various online specialist stores. They are not typically seen on the high street or in general retail and are still considered the preserve of professionals. Unlike kinesiology tape and massage tools, which have recently become popular to try at home, non-professionals are not very likely to try cupping without professional guidance.

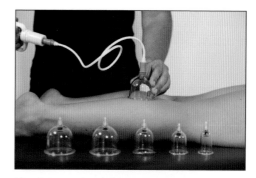

Figure 2.1. A set of vacuum-pump cups

The most popular cupping sets are the plastic-cup and vacuum-pump kits, which usually come as a set of different-sized cups with a hand pump to create the vacuum (figure 2.1). I would recommend getting a set of these, and I use them throughout this book.

You will notice I commonly use RockPods throughout this book (figure 2.2)—they are a type of silicone cup from the RockTape brand. As part of my work, I teach a very popular course on the use of RockPods.

Glass cups (figure 2.3) will either have a rubber bulb attached to the top to create

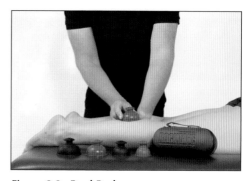

Figure 2.2. RockPods

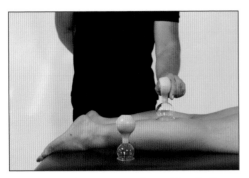

Figure 2.3. Glass cups with a rubber bulb

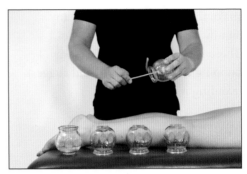

Figure 2.4. Glass cups with a flame

the vacuum or require a flame to create a vacuum within the cup just prior to application (figure 2.4). Glass cups have a quality feel to them, with smooth, beveled edges around the cup's rim. They are not suitable for the movement-based interventions covered in this book. Essentially—glass breaks!

There are also some more high-tech cups arriving on the market to service the increased demand for cupping therapy. Companies such as Achedaway have developed a battery-operated, pulsing cup that creates and maintains its own variable vacuum (figure 2.5).

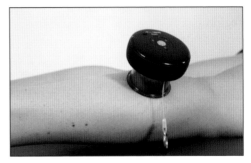

Figure 2.5. Achedaway's battery-operated cup

An overview of some of the different vacuum cups available is outlined in the following table.

Different Types of Vacuum Cups			
Cup Design	**Vacuum Mechanism**	**Benefits**	**Limitations**
Manual plastic valved cups	Manual hand pump	• Easy to adjust vacuum • Cheap to buy • Easy to see the skin condition inside the cups	• Difficult to clean around the valves • Easy to create excessive vacuum

(Continued)

Different Types of Vacuum Cups			
Cup Design	**Vacuum Mechanism**	**Benefits**	**Limitations**
Silicone cups, e.g. RockPods	Deformation and reformation of the cups	• Can be applied quickly • Inexpensive • Softer edges • Easy to clean • Will not break if dropped	• Unable to see the skin inside the pod • Too soft for glide cupping
Glass vacuum cups (with bulb)	Rubber bulb attached to the top of the glass cup	• Easy to apply • Smooth edge around the rim	• Not suitable for active movement-based interventions due to fragility of the glass
Glass vacuum cups (no bulb)	Flame	• Smooth but firm edges are good for glide cupping	• Risk of burns and fire • Increased insurance premium
Automatic vacuum cups, e.g. Achedaway Cupper	Automatic	• Easy for self-application • Can offer pulsatile vacuum • Novel experience	• Difficult to customize the vacuum pressure • More complex to use • Expensive

Demonstration of different cups in use

hypoallergenic materials such as glass, plastic, and silicone, the introduction of oil-based lubricants may pose a risk to patients with sensitive skin or allergies. Make sure you ask your patients if they have any known allergies. For example, a nut allergy would preclude the use of any nut-based waxes and oils.

Using Oils, Creams, and Waxes

Using a form of lubricant can help to secure the seal between the edge of the cup and the skin. Lubricant will also be needed if you wish to glide the cups along the skin. While cups are made from

If you are aiming for the cup to fix on the skin and not glide, so that it creates a fixed handle for soft-tissue mobilization, then I recommend applying only a thin layer of wax or oil around the rim of the cup to help secure a good vacuum but prevent the cup from sliding over the skin.

If you wish for the cup to glide more freely with patient movement or with a more passive glide mechanism, you will need to cover the body region with a suitable lubricant (wax, oil, or cream) prior to cupping.

Top Tip

If you are applying oils to the skin in preparation for cupping, I would recommend washing your hands after the oil application and before cupping so that you can more readily grip the cups. You will find this practice rather essential when using glass cups, as these become very slippery and difficult to grip if they have oil on them. Some practitioners wear a medical glove when applying oil so they do not need to wash their hands as frequently.

Working with Body Hair

Perhaps unsurprisingly, cupping over hairy areas can be difficult, and, in some cases, just not possible. If you are struggling to get your cups to adhere to hairy skin, try some oil, cream, or wax first. You may also wish to experiment with different sizes of cups or different materials and vacuum methods. In some cases, it may not be possible to secure a cup in place, so be prepared to concede in some circumstances.

How Long Should You Cup For?

Traditionally, cups are left in place for 5 to 20 minutes. Even after 5 minutes, the residual markings are often significant and can last for a few weeks. Although rarely harmful, in Western cultures these markings are commonly undesirable, although not always. Fortunately, it is possible to achieve the therapeutic benefits of cupping with much shorter time frames of 2 minutes or less, and even a few seconds can be very therapeutic when combined with active or passive movement.

Applying the Cups

Valved Cups

Place the cup over the skin and attach the vacuum pump. Begin to create a vacuum by squeezing the hand pump (figure 2.6). Ask the patient to report any discomfort during the procedure. The aim is to create a suitable vacuum that allows you to move the cup without

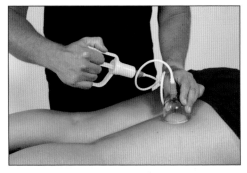

Figure 2.6. Simple application of a plastic vacuum pump

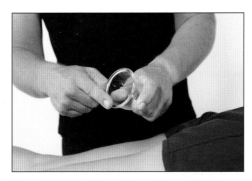

Figure 2.7. Running a fingertip around the edge of a cup to check for rough edges

breaking the seal and losing the vacuum, while providing a therapeutic level of skin tension not deemed uncomfortable by the patient. This is very variable between individuals.

Valved cups perform best for passive and glide cupping treatments. Always check that the rim of the cup is smooth and free from any rough edges that may damage the skin. This is easily achieved by running your fingertip around the edge of the cup prior to application (figure 2.7).

It is possible to use plastic valved cups for the active cupping techniques, but I prefer to use softer silicone cups because they can deform during movement, which has the benefit of modulating the vacuum and avoiding an excessive level of vacuum being created by the patient's movement.

Silicone Cups

Silicone cups create a vacuum by reforming their shape following a manual compression. They may fail to fully

reshape or may deform during treatment if a high level of vacuum is created. Silicone cups are ideal for beginners and the best option for self-cupping techniques.

To apply a silicone cup, squash the top of the cup down to deform it. With the RockPods, this can be achieved with three levels of compression (figure 2.8).

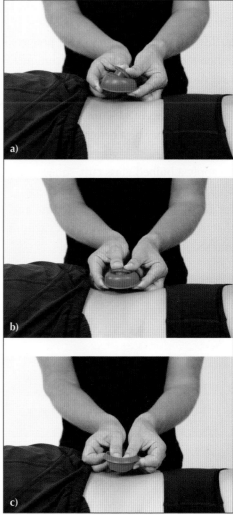

Figure 2.8. Different levels of compression with RockPods: (a) semi compressed; (b) full compression; (c) inverted

Once compressed, affix the cup to the skin. Some emollient may be required. Release the cup with the rim sealed onto the skin, and allow the reshaping of the cup to create the vacuum. The cup is then ready to perform the techniques outlined in the following chapters.

Glass Cups with Bulbs

The smooth, beveled edges of good-quality glass cups make them the preferred option for most glide cupping techniques. I say most, because over more-contoured areas of the body the rigid edge of the cup may cause a loss of vacuum, and a softer silicone cup may be a better option.

To apply a bulbed glass cup, squeeze the bulb, place the cup in position, check for an effective seal around the rim, and then release the bulb to create a vacuum and secure the cup (figure 2.9).

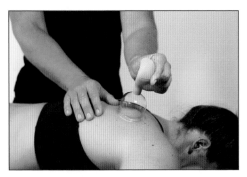

Figure 2.9. Application of a bulbed glass cup

Glass Cups (Fire Cupping)

Glass cups, one of the more traditional types of cup, require a flame to create

a vacuum within the cup. When the correct equipment is used, the method of application is not as dangerous as many non-practitioners assume. However, it will push your professional insurance cost up and does take more training time to reach a safe level of competency. Perhaps unsurprisingly, it is not generally considered a suitable self-management strategy.

To perform a fire cupping application, first make sure your patient is in a relaxed and stable position. Do not ask your patient to move or stretch when using glass cups. Apply a base layer of oil or wax to the body region you are going to cup. Wash your hands and make sure the glass cups do not have oil on them—you do not want to be handling a naked flame while attempting to grip slippery cups with oily fingers.

Take a cupping igniter—a metal stick with a cotton-wool ball at one end—and dip the cotton end in a 70–90% alcohol solution. In my experience, the lower-percentage solutions will create a lower level of vacuum. Light the alcohol-doused cotton ball with a lighter operable with one hand and briefly place it inside a glass cup while holding the cup at a downward angle (figure 2.10). The flame should be placed fully inside the cup and then removed as one continuous motion. Do not hold the flame inside the cup.

As soon as the flame is removed, place the cup directly onto the patient's skin. Once in place, the cups have

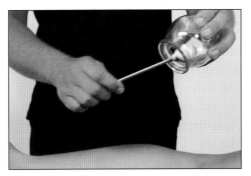

Figure 2.10. Light the alcohol-doused cotton ball and briefly place it inside a glass cup held at a downward angle

traditionally been left for a few minutes without any further manipulation. Depending on patient comfort, often in direct proportion to the level of vacuum created, I would recommend mobilizing the cups or trying some glide cupping.

Essentially, fire cupping is just a more extravagant method of creating a vacuum. The result is a cup with a vacuum that you can then mobilize. Remember that patient movement is not advisable with glass cups.

Different cup applications

Safety Tips

Following the fire-cupping application, information in this book will not allow you to become trained, competent,

or insured in the use of fire cupping. Spending time with a trained professional, being assessed, and receiving competency certification is required. I hope you can appreciate the legal requirement for me to write this caveat and my personal desire to avoid any harm to your patients and your reputation. The following safety guidelines are recommended.

1. Make sure flammable materials are kept at a safe distance from the flame and treatment area.
2. Have some water, a wet cloth, and a fire extinguisher in the room with you. Hopefully you will not need these.
3. Hold the cup over the patient in your dominant hand, and hold the fire stick in your non-dominant hand away from the patient.
4. Keep the flame away from your patient.
5. Do not keep the flame in the cup; this will heat the cup, which could burn your patient. The flame should be placed in the cup and then immediately removed.

Removing the Cups

To remove a cup, gently lift and tilt it (figure 2.11) while applying counter-pressure down onto the skin with one finger or thumb. The aim is to break the seal at one specific point, which will eliminate the vacuum with minimal added skin strain. Silicone cups can be squeezed to deform the cup and reduce

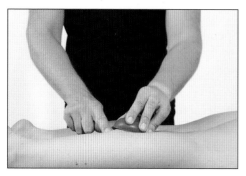

Figure 2.11. Gently lift and tilt the cup with some counter-pressure to break the seal

the vacuum. Valved cups may have the option to release the valve, and bulbed cups can be removed by squeezing the bulb to reduce the vacuum. Do not remove cups by simply pulling them.

Cleaning and Sanitizing

Most cups can be easily cleaned using antibacterial or antimicrobial soap and water. Be careful if using stronger clinical disinfectant wipes, as they can cause the breakdown of silicone cups. The use of wipes does not offer the same debris-washout mechanism of soap and water rinsing. Once the cups have been cleaned, ensure they are effectively dried using disposable paper towels and air drying as required. Ensure no moisture remains inside any of the cups, bulbs, or valve mechanisms.

The Mechanics of Cupping

Understanding the Biomechanics of Cupping

As discussed in chapter 1, cupping is an ancient medical treatment. Like many traditional treatments, its long history is embedded with doctrine and folk wisdom. Tradition and science are not usually aligned, thus there is little demand for an evidence base or the identification of a biologically plausible mechanism. In this chapter we will review some of the findings from an excellent research paper by Tham, Lee, and Lu (2006), who studied cupping from a biomechanical perspective, and in doing so shed some light on the biomechanics of cupping therapy.

The unique feature of cupping is the vacuum, and the distinct feeling of skin tension that it creates, and in this chapter we will focus on the science that explains the scale and distribution of the tensile and compressive forces that accompany this therapeutic modality.

Contact between the cup and the skin creates a ring of compression directly under the rim of the cup (figure 3.1).

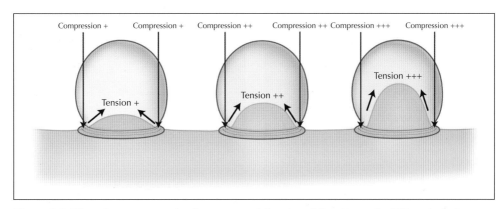

Figure 3.1. There is a compressive force around the rim of the cup and a lifting strain force that domes the skin beneath and within the cup

Most solid cups have rolled edges, and the softer silicone cups have a flat edge to disperse this compressive force. A vacuum device with a sharper rim would cause a higher compressive force and be a potential cause of discomfort. It is important to remember when applying cups to painful regions that although the cup lifts the skin, it does so by compressing the skin underneath its perimeter edge. Care should be taken to ensure a comfortable placement or to utilize a sufficiently wide cup that spans over a painful region.

We often refer to the skin within the cup as undergoing decompression as it is sucked up into the cup. This is supported by simple ultrasonography tests, which show increases in the subcutaneous space (figure 3.2). It is important to understand how this decompression occurs and the tensile nature of the physical stress it places on the tissues beneath the skin, which include the fragile capillary network. The tensile stress on the capillaries causes the reddening (ecchymosis) that we witness following sustained or high-vacuum applications (see also chapter 4).

Tham et al. (2006) noted that the tensile stress occurs mostly in the mid-portion of the cup and extends down to the muscle layer. The maximum tensile stress on the skin occurs just inside the rim of the cup as a result of the skin being both anchored by the rim and stretched up into the cup by the vacuum. This helps to explain the pattern of ecchymosis seen after cupping: a reddening that usually begins in a ringlike pattern before filling the center of the circle (figure 3.3).

It appears that the tissue tension from cupping does not extend beyond the area enclosed by the cup. However, this finding relates to static cupping and does not consider the movement of the cups while they are fixed on the skin. This shearing style of treatment is likely to broaden the distribution of the tensile stress through the skin (figure 3.4).

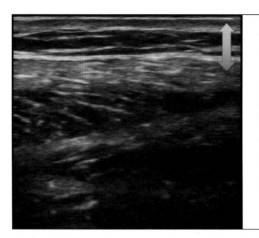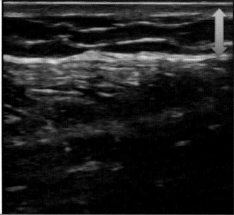

Figure 3.2. The subcutaneous space with and without cupping

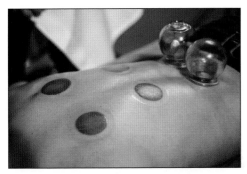

Figure 3.3. The ecchymosis seen after cupping is reddening that usually begins as a ring and later fills in

The skin under the rim of the cup remains under a compressive load, which will not cause capillary rupture. Reddening of the skin may occur under the rim of the cup following repeated twisting, which could create a damaging level of friction between the cup and the skin and should be avoided.

While some traditional teachings suggest that smaller cups will produce a deeper effect, research indicates the opposite is true, with wider cups achieving a deeper transmission of tensile force in comparison to smaller cups for any given vacuum pressure.

An understanding of the biomechanics of cupping helps us to deliver comfortable and effective treatment sessions by recognizing the potential discomfort caused by excessive compression under the rim of the cup. The selection of a suitably sized cup and avoiding friction between the skin and the rim of the cup are also advisable strategies to ensure patient comfort.

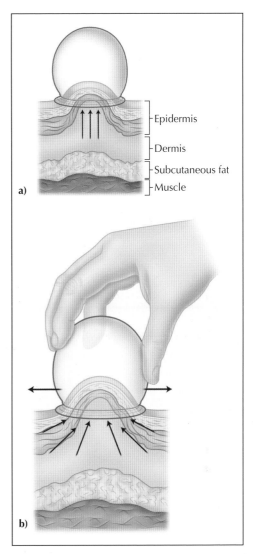

Figure 3.4. (a) Tissue tension with static cupping is contained beneath the cup; (b) when the cup is moved, the tissue tension broadens and becomes more radial

Reference

Tham, L. M., H. P. Lee, and C. Lu. 2006. "Cupping: From a biomechanical perspective." *Journal of Biomechanics* 39(12): 2183–93.

The Physiology of Cupping

Understanding the Circular Markings

The markings left by cupping (figure 4.1) are commonly referred to as bruises, but this description is debatable. The term "bruise" is probably used because of the lack of a more suitable descriptive and explanatory word, but bruising is not typically associated with a therapeutic response. I am also not comfortable with the term "therapeutic bruising" for the temporary markings following cupping because it's difficult to consider bruising as therapeutic.

A bruise is often defined as an injury associated with skin discoloration and pain. Cupping may cause the type of discoloration that is associated with a bruise, but it is not caused by injury or impact, and the marking is not usually painful.

The discoloration can be described as "ecchymosis" or "erythema," but

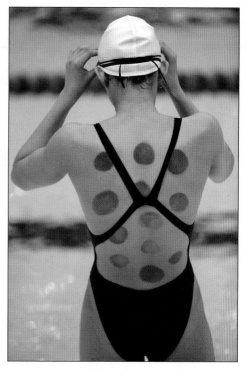

Figure 4.1. An athlete showing cupping marks
Image © Getty Images

these are not patient-friendly words to pronounce. I would suggest using the simple terms "markings" or "blemishes" as they are words most patients are familiar with, and they are not associated with injury in the same way that bruises are.

Why Do the Markings Look like Bruises?

Bruising in healthy people is usually caused by a rapid impact that ruptures the small blood vessels under the skin. This causes blood to spread from the damaged blood vessels and create a patch of discolored skin, which usually changes color over time as the blood cells are metabolized as part of the immune response.

The discoloration from cupping occurs in much the same way, except with low force and prolonged tissue stress. That is to say that it is a gentler force held over a longer period of time and without the initial trauma that causes

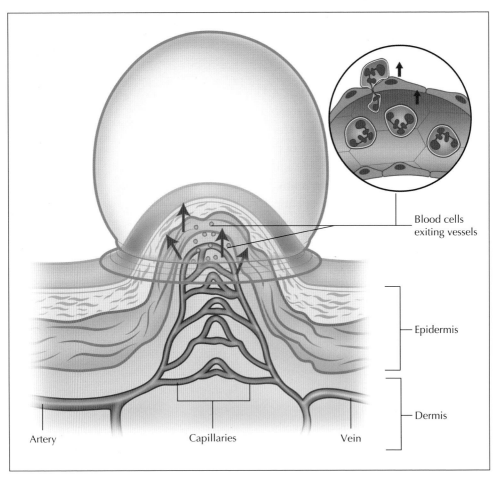

Blood cells exiting vessels

Epidermis

Dermis

Artery   Capillaries   Vein

Figure 4.2. The vacuum pulls the skin up into the cup, causing the delicate micro-capillaries to stretch, rupture, and dilate

the discoloration associated with a bruise.

The Physiology of Cupping

The vacuum pulls the skin up into the cup, which stresses the delicate micro-capillaries and causes them to stretch, rupture, or dilate (figure 4.2). If the capillaries dilate, they allow the seepage of blood into surrounding tissues while the vessel walls remain intact. This is called *diapedesis* and is typically associated with an inflammatory immune response. The rupture or dilation of the capillaries causes the typical pattern of discoloration seen during and after the removal of a vacuum cup.

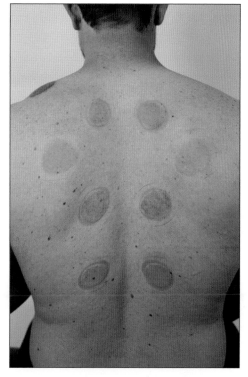

Figure 4.4. Ecchymosis from cupping

The reddening of the skin can be described as *erythema* (figure 4.3). A darker purple discoloration is termed *ecchymosis* (figure 4.4), and small red spots are called *petechiae* (figure 4.5). If a vacuum remains for too long, *purpura* (figure 4.6) may occur from prolonged hemorrhaging of blood vessels beneath the skin, and blisters may also occur. Both of these responses can be avoided by using a low vacuum pressure and a short duration of application.

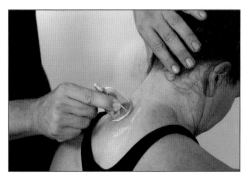

Figure 4.3. Erythema from cupping

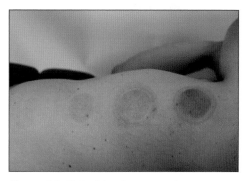

Figure 4.5. Petechiae from cupping

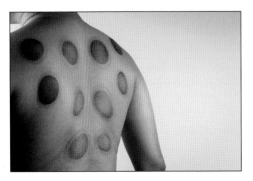

Figure 4.6. Purpura from cupping

Immune Response

The capillary stress and erythema cause an increase in cellular activity that may offer an anti-inflammatory and pain-reducing effect.

Lowe (2017) discussed how the immune response to the capillary rupture includes the digestion of degraded blood cells by specialized cells called macrophages. This cellular response triggers the production of the enzyme heme oxygenase 1, which breaks down the heme from the hemoglobin. The breakdown of the heme results in the production of carbon monoxide, biliverdin, and bilirubin, which have been shown to have antioxidant, anti-inflammatory, and neuromodulatory properties.

Summary: Cupping Marks

Post-cupping marks on the skin are often incorrectly labelled bruises. Their appearance can be explained using a knowledge of the vascular response to the tissue strain created by the vacuum within the cups. The increased activity of cells with immune function following capillary rupture provides a positive healing environment around injured soft tissue and mediates nociceptive (perception of pain or injury) input.

While the discoloration associated with cupping may be explained as a positive effect, the modern approach to cupping seeks to minimize the discoloration in favor of a more neurosensory mechanism.

Cupping and Blood Flow

Explaining the Effects of Cupping on Blood Flow

Cupping practitioners often claim that cupping improves blood flow and refer to the circular reddening of the skin as clear evidence for this. We can learn more about blood flow within the micro-environment of the vacuum from a fascinating photoacoustic imaging study on the ear of a mouse (Zhou et al. 2020). I do not think the mouse was harmed during this experiment, and if you are wondering why a mouse had to be used in the first place, it was because of the thinness of its ear, as the monitoring system used to detect changes in blood flow after cupping works only to a depth of 1 mm.

In the experiment, a low-level vacuum was applied to the mouse's ear for 5 minutes, and images were taken of the pattern of blood flow afterward.

The results are clear to see: compared to the pre-cupping images, the post-cupping images show a 64% increase in blood vessel density. More blood is also seen in the existing blood vessels, represented by a higher intensity image (figure 4.7). However, this increased blood is reported to be congested within the capillaries and cannot therefore be described in such simple terms as faster blood flow.

The images also show a patch of capillary blood perfusion, or micro-bleeding. This is thought to be the cause of the typical clinical presentation of superficial reddening witnessed after cupping treatment.

The increased vascularization increases the oxygen utilization within

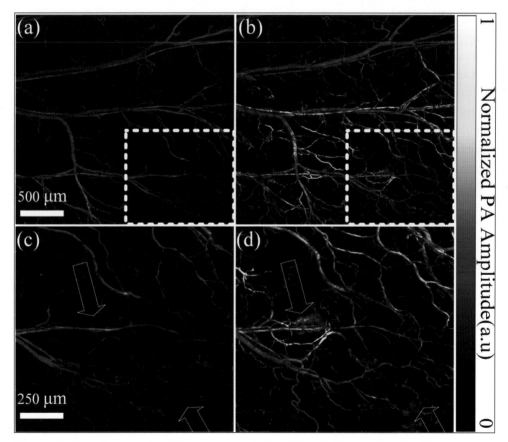

Figure 4.7. Vascular content of the mouse ear before (a) and after cupping (b); (c) shows a close-up of the dashed box in (a), and (d) a close-up of the dashed box in (b), with arrows labelling perfusion (image reproduced from Zhou et al. [2020])

both the vacuumed and adjacent tissues and therefore represents a short-term increase in local metabolism that dissipates once the vacuum is removed. It is not possible to ascertain how long these changes last after the removal of the vacuum, but as with the discoloration we see on the skin, it may be determined by the duration and strength of the vacuum application.

enough evidence to determine such a "sweet spot," but there is evidence of the harm caused by excessive and prolonged vacuum cupping, indicating that a minimal-dose approach is probably the best way to start.

The minimal-dose concept is one of the defining principles that allows the safe and effective use of cupping in a modern manual-therapy context.

Conclusion: Cupping and Blood Flow

I believe it is logical to assume that the increased vascularization and perfusion that occurred within the mouse's ear in this study are representative of the vascular changes that occur in humans. The extent of these changes is probably linked to vacuum intensity and duration, and therefore it may be reasonable to assume that a therapeutic optimum exists for each of these factors. There is not yet

References

Lowe, D. T. 2017. "Cupping therapy: An analysis of the effects of suction on skin and the possible influence on human health." *Complementary Therapies in Clinical Practice* 29: 162–68.

Zhou, Y., F. Cao, H. Li, X. Huang, D. Wei, L. Wang, and P. Lai. 2020. "Photoacoustic imaging of micro-environmental changes in facial cupping therapy." *Biomedical Optics Express* 11(5): 2394–2401.

Cupping and the Nervous System

Understanding How the Nervous System Responds
to Cupping Therapy

Introduction

Like all other manual therapies, cupping provides a sensory input to the brain. The unique sensation of skin strain created by the vacuum is rapidly communicated through the peripheral nervous system to the central nervous system, where the sensation is perceived, and the brain can then respond. For example, if you create too much vacuum over a sensitive area, then the patient may feel pain and limit their movement in an attempt to reduce skin strain under the cup.

If the cups are placed carefully and are comfortable, then the patient will hopefully experience pain relief and be encouraged to move more as a result. The response to cupping can vary significantly between patients and is dependent on the way a person's nervous system responds to the unique feeling of an applied vacuum. The factors influencing this individual response might include culture, expectation, and treatment setting.

Understanding Pain Relief

One of the most popular scientific explanations for pain relief is the "pain-gate theory" proposed by Ronald Melzack and Patrick Wall in 1965 (figure 5.1). The theory proposes that when a non-painful tactile stimulation, such as massage, is applied to a perceived painful area, we experience pain relief in that specific body location. This theory may explain the phenomenon of rubbing a sore spot where an injury has just occurred. Cupping over a painful area may reduce pain via this pain-gate mechanism.

Since the publication of Melzack and Wall's theory in 1965, the study of pain has snowballed into a research specialism of considerable size, and the prevailing opinion is that the most

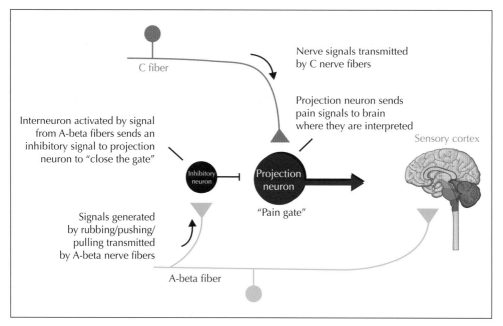

Figure 5.1. The pain-gate theory

robust pain-management framework is the biopsychosocial approach (figure 5.2). The question of whether cupping reduces pain is perhaps too simplistic and we should instead ask: How can cupping fit into a modern approach to pain management?

Modern pain management requires patients, clinicians, and their social support networks to recognize the complexity of pain. This is no easy task in the modern world, where so many things can be "fixed" or replaced with minimal effort. Any patient who is suffering from one of the many causes of musculoskeletal pain would likely report a positive pain-relieving response from the passive and active techniques outlined within this book. For many, even short-term pain relief would be a satisfactory outcome. This book

aims to offer the clinician the option of more advanced cupping methods that more closely align with modern manual therapy and pain-management strategies.

For example, explaining pain to patients has become a key component of modern treatment. Many of us have at least a moderate level of confidence in our ability to explain pain, but we fail to consider the nonverbal, movement-mediated pain education we may be providing when we combine a manual therapy like cupping with movement. A specific example could be cupping over the lumbar spine. The therapeutic sensory stimulus of the cups, combined with guided movement of the lumbar spine, not only encourages a "stiff" patient to start moving but also provides a learning experience that pain can be

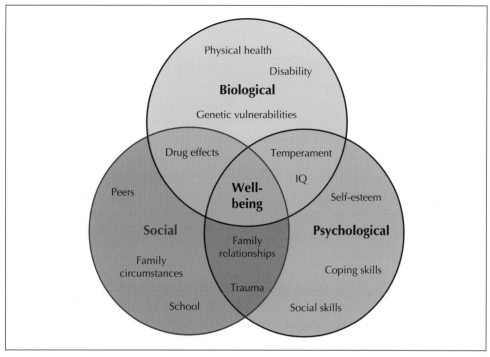

Figure 5.2. The biopsychosocial approach to well-being

managed and movement can occur without harm, reducing the fear of movement that confines so many of our patients.

In addition, as highlighted in this chapter, the sensory stimulus from cupping can improve feedback to the brain, which is especially important when pain and reduced use have started to negatively influence the awareness and control of that region. By harnessing the analgesic and mechano-stimulating effects of cupping and combining them with movement and education within a supportive and therapeutic setting, you will offer your patients a more robust biopsychosocial treatment that supports a longer-term self-management approach, thus fitting in with the modern approach to manual therapy and pain management.

It is worth noting how acupuncture has been accepted as a pain-management tool in many health-care systems. Although acupuncture and cupping look and feel very different, when you consider their history and passive method of delivery, there are identified similarities.

Encouraging Movement

When we ask patients to move and stretch an area of their body for rehabilitation purposes, it is likely that they feel only the intense sensations associated with moving into end-range positions, which may be reduced due to reported pain and muscle sensitivity. This is normal and reflects the nervous system's inbuilt but variable thresholds for the detection of stress and strain within the tissues. Within the mid-range of most movements, people do not typically feel any notable sensation. The addition of one or more cups to standard joint movement can significantly increase the sensory feedback and create more stimulus during normal movement.

When I am teaching, I feel this is more readily experienced than explained. I always do my best to articulate the concept of increased feedback, but when students experience this method of active cupping, they are immediately aware of the benefits. The neck and lower back are particular beneficiaries of this augmented movement approach. Patients often describe it as feeling like a self-massage or an enhanced stretch.

The control of motion is partially determined by proprioception—that is, the awareness of the position and movement of the body. Proprioception is often negatively affected by pain, and some areas of our body naturally have a lower level of proprioception, such as the trunk and the shoulder blades. Just think how challenging it can be to teach scapulothoracic or pelvic-control exercises to patients.

Proprioception can be restored or improved with exercises that focus on technique and control. Movement control can be enhanced by increasing the available feedback to the brain, which aids the feedback and correction loops that exist within the motor control system. The sustained skin-strain stimulus created by the vacuum within the cup provides a quick and practical way to restore movement function by increasing proprioception through the enhanced awareness of that body region.

Smudging and Correcting Sensory Input

For the reader looking for a little bit more neuroscience, in this next section I will attempt to explain the theory of smudging, the correction of cortical representation, and what this may have to do with cupping.

Smudging is a term that refers to the disruption of neural body representations in the brain's somatosensory cortex. Pain and reduced movement can cause a reduced sensory and motor accuracy, with resulting reductions in movement control and mismatches between sensory input and motor output that are often associated with pain. Research indicates that disrupted body representations can be corrected with the help of sensory discrimination training. This is because paying attention to, and differentiating between, different sensory inputs can help correct the smudging and lead to a more favorable analgesic outcome (Moseley et al. 2008). This approach makes for interesting reading, but how can we apply it in the practice of cupping?

The delivery of a manual stimulus such as massage or mobilization is usually interpreted as either therapeutic or nontherapeutic, and patients rarely concentrate on the stimulus other than to enjoy the overall experience, or wish for it to end! This may be because the treatment is delivered in a nonspecific way or the patient has no reason or motive to focus on the stimulus, which in many cases is delivered in a dulled manner to avoid applying too much focused pressure over tender areas.

Think of a typical lower-back massage, performed with the palms of the hands over the lumbar region while encouraging the patient to relax. This style of treatment is proven, and we know it is likely to help our patients; what I am suggesting here is that by getting patients to pay more attention to a passive sensory stimulus, we may be able to better support the correction of the smudged body representations that can occur following injury and continued dysfunction.

Cupping is an excellent way of delivering sensory discrimination training, and examples are shown below for the lumbar spine, upper back, and neck (figures 5.3–5.5).

Sensory Discrimination Training with Vacuum Cups

Example of discrimation training

Place six cups over the lumbar spine and draw a labeled representation of these for the patient to see during treatment (figure 5.3). As you perform active, passive, or a combination of both cupping treatments, ask the patient to give feedback on which cups they feel are being mobilized. Make sure you tell the patient if there are any errors in their sensory perception so they can begin to correct them during this exercise.

This concept can also be utilized for the upper back (figure 5.4) and the neck (figure 5.5).

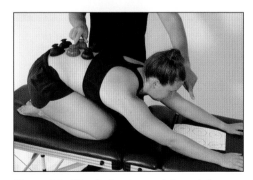

Figure 5.3 Discrimination training of the lumbar spine

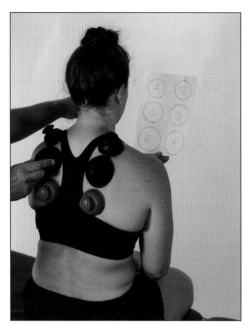

Figure 5.4. Discrimination training of the upper back

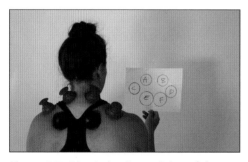

Figure 5.5. Discrimination training of the neck

Conclusion

The past decade has seen a steady shift in people's understanding of manual therapy, from the earlier mechanical understanding to a more-recent consideration of the influence manual therapy has on the nervous system. Cupping should not be exempt from this paradigm shift; however, many recent cupping texts and scientific studies examining the use of cupping pay little or no attention to the involvement of the nervous system. This may explain why cupping has not been so rapidly accepted by Western medical practitioners. When you consider the valuable input that cupping may offer the nervous system, the use of this style of manual therapy can take its place among the already-accepted treatments and assist with the modern approach to injury and pain management.

Reference

Moseley, G. L., N. M. Zalucki, and K. Wiech. 2008. "Tactile discrimination, but not tactile stimulation alone, reduces chronic limb pain." *Pain* 137: 600–608.

Cupping for the Foot, Ankle, and Lower Leg

How to Use Cupping Techniques in the Management of Foot, Ankle, and Lower-Leg Pain

Introduction

Beginning underneath the foot, plantar fasciitis, or plantar heel pain, is a common condition that is typically stubborn in response to therapeutic interventions. The prevalence rates of plantar heel pain are higher among athletes, runners, and the over-fifties (Lopes et al. 2012; Thomas et al. 2019). The onset of plantar heel pain is often gradual and related to occupation, body weight, or exercise training. This makes curing the condition challenging. Passive pain-relieving interventions like cupping, taping, self-massage, and percussion tools are very helpful for pain management, alongside more exercise-based strategies.

Moving up to the ankle, the most common injury at this joint is the twisted ankle, or inversion injury. Rehabilitation following an inversion soft-tissue injury requires the restoration of balance, strength, range of motion, and a normal gait pattern. We can use the neurosensory input from cupping to augment our rehabilitation plans following ankle injury.

My students and I have had some success in the use of cupping around the Achilles tendon, where you can often achieve a surprising level of vacuum over the medial and lateral sides of the lower tendon. This offers a pain-relieving mechanism as part of a passive or part-active intervention, shown within this chapter.

Cupping is very easy to use around the calf region for the management of pain and tension and to augment stretching routines. I have also used it in the management of anterior compartment syndrome, and I will show these techniques shortly.

Getting Started

This chapter aims to show you how to use dry cupping safely and effectively around the foot, ankle, and lower leg. A full assessment should be performed before beginning any cupping treatment, and the presence of any contraindications would preclude the use of cupping therapy.

Using the standard application principles outlined in chapter 2, begin with the patient in a comfortable position based on the area you wish to treat. This is typically face down, or prone, with the feet off the end of the couch or with the knee flexed (figure 6.1).

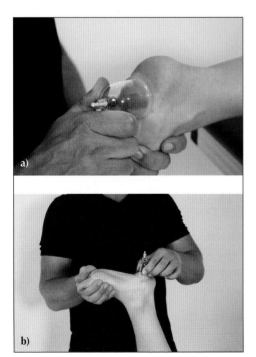

Figure 6.1. Prone position with cups in situ (a) with feet off the end of the couch and (b) with knee bent and foot up

Foot Techniques

Before you attempt to apply one or more cups to the sole of the foot, make sure the plantar skin is clean and then liberally apply some wax or oil to enhance the seal around the edge of the cup. On occasion, it may not be possible to achieve or sustain a suitable vacuum on the foot; if you have tried and failed with different types of cup and applied oil or wax, then it may just be due to skin tension or foot shape and not clinician error.

Passive Cupping for the Foot

Begin with the patient in a relaxed position, with the sole of the foot easily accessible and free to move so you can flex or extend the foot to alter the plantar skin tension to help secure a good vacuum.

Apply one cup with a moderate level of vacuum over the sole of the foot. If the application causes an increase in pain, remove the cup and try relocating it. Using a lower level of vacuum pressure may also help. Following the successful application of the cup, use one hand to mobilize the cup and underlying soft tissue, while the other hand holds and stabilizes the foot (figure 6.2). Increasing the vacuum pressure will allow the delivery of a more vigorous passive mobilization if desirable.

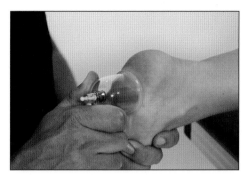

Figure 6.2. Passive single-foot application

While it may be possible to apply two or more cups to the sole of the foot at the same time, I would recommend applying just one and then repositioning it so that cups are not in situ without being mobilized.

Receiving cupping therapy on the soles of your feet has been described as one of life's greatest pleasures—judge for yourself by having someone perform cupping on your own feet.

Active Cupping for the Foot

With one or more cups over the sole of the foot, instruct the patient to flex and extend their foot in combination with ankle dorsiflexion and plantar flexion. With this technique, it is common for the cups to fall off as the significant changes in skin tension cause the seal to break around the perimeter of the cup, leading to a loss of vacuum. For this reason, as with other active techniques, I would recommend using softer cups, such as the silicone RockPods used in figure 6.3.

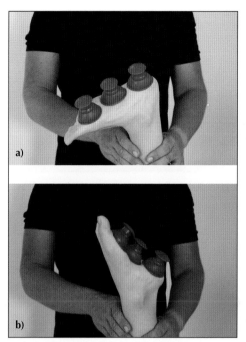

a)

b)

Figure 6.3. Using RockPods on the foot with (a) active dorsiflexion and (b) plantar flexion

Cupping the foot with plastic cup and then silicone active cupping

Glide Cupping for the Foot

This technique can be difficult to achieve with some patients. Remember to make sure the foot is clean and oiled or waxed before applying a suitably sized rigid cup that can glide up or down the sole of the foot (figure 6.4).

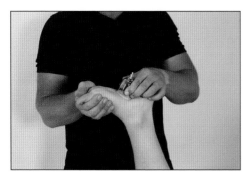

Figure 6.4. Glide cupping on the sole of the foot

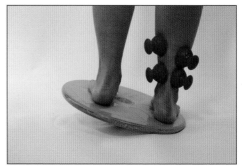

Figure 6.5. Placement of cups around the ankle and lower leg during a balance exercise on a balance board

Ankle Techniques

The ankle techniques differ from the plantar-foot techniques by utilizing the neurosensory benefits of cupping to augment exercise rehabilitation, whereas on the foot they were used for more direct soft-tissue mobilization and pain relief.

The following techniques are recommended to sit alongside an evidence-based ankle-inversion-sprain rehabilitation program, where the four main aims are:

1. Restoration of balance
2. Regaining ankle range of motion
3. Restoration of ankle strength
4. Normalizing the gait pattern.

Restoration of Balance

Our balance, when standing on one leg for example, is maintained by three inputs: visual, vestibular (inner ear), and proprioceptive. Proprioception refers to the sensations from the joints, muscles, and skin that help the brain to calibrate our position. We can use the cup vacuum to increase skin tension, which provides an increased proprioceptive stimulus and reduces the thresholds of stimulation from motion and skin stretch. I would explain this to the patient as the cups making the brain more aware of the ankle and therefore aiding control and balance (figure 6.5).

Regaining Ankle Range of Motion

Ankle inversion injuries often cause a significant loss of ankle-joint mobility. Dorsiflexion is the most important ankle motion for normal walking and running, and regaining this motion is often the focus of ankle manual-therapy techniques. You cannot use cups to mobilize the talocrural joint, but they

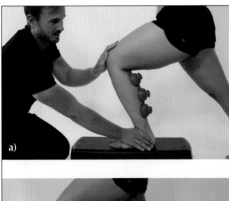

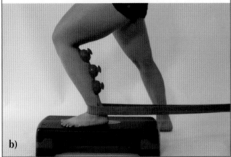

Figure 6.6. Lunge dorsiflexion with (a) hands-on mobilization with cups over posterior calf and (b) mobility band plus cups

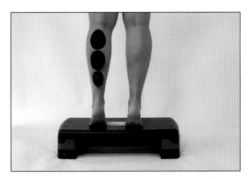

Figure 6.7. Strengthening exercise with pods on calf

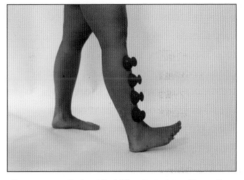

Figure 6.8. Gait-rehabilitation exercise using RockPods

may help to create some soft-tissue shearing over the calf region during dorsiflexion mobilization and stretching exercises. An example is shown in figure 6.6.

Ankle Strengthening and Normalizing the Gait Pattern

The sensory stimulation from the cups may help to improve movement awareness during strengthening (figure 6.7) and gait-rehabilitation exercises (figure 6.8).

Ankle on wobble board, lunges, lunges with band, calf raises, dorsiflexion into gait re-education

Cupping for Achilles-Tendon Pain

Load management is the typical focus of Achilles-tendon pain treatment, but passive interventions that reduce

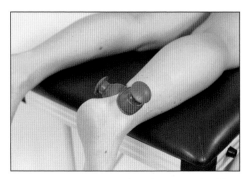

Figure 6.9. Two cups placed, one each side of the Achilles tendon

pain and tension are well received by patients. Even if the therapeutic techniques provide only transient relief, the experience offers a positive treatment outcome and indicates the likelihood of further recovery. We have experimented in clinic and on courses with the location of the cups and have found that it is often possible to achieve a vacuum to the sides of the Achilles tendon cord (figure 6.9).

In cases where this is not possible, you will find that the cups will be more

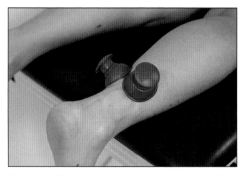

Figure 6.10. Two cups placed, one each side of the Achilles tendon slightly higher up the leg

easily applied slightly higher up the leg (figure 6.10).

Passive Achilles Cupping

Once in place, the cups can be passively mobilized to provide a gentle soft-tissue mobilization around the tendon (figure 6.11).

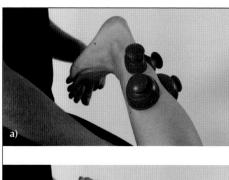

Figure 6.11. Passive Achilles cupping

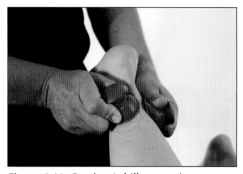

a)

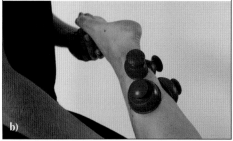

b)

Figure 6.12. Active Achilles cupping with (a) dorsiflexion and (b) plantar flexion

Active Achilles Cupping

With the cups in situ to the sides of the tendon, the patient can be instructed to dorsiflex and plantar flex the ankle to create an active stretching and shearing effect (figure 6.12).

Passive and active Achilles

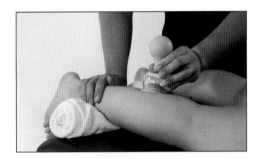

Figure 6.13. Passive gastroc-soleus position with patient prone, feet off the end of the couch, rolled-up towel under the ankles, one cup on the mid-calf, and one hand stabilizing the ankle

Cupping the Gastrocnemius and Soleus

Cupping the back of the lower leg over the gastrocnemius and soleus is easy to perform and well received by patients. It is often a good area to introduce cupping to patients and a good region to begin practicing in the use of cups. It is worth reiterating that you should not cup over a deep vein thrombosis (DVT) and that the lower leg is the most common site for a DVT. The symptoms of this include swelling, heat, reddening, and pain. People with a suspected DVT should report to an emergency medical department and should not receive any form of manual therapy.

Passive Gastroc-Soleus Techniques

Begin with the patient lying prone with the feet projecting off the end of the treatment couch. You may wish to place a cushion or rolled-up towel under the shin to shorten the gastrocnemius. I recommend using just one cup to allow the other hand to stabilize the leg as you mobilize the cup, which in turn mobilizes the underlying soft tissue (figure 6.13).

Active Gastroc-Soleus Techniques

Begin with the patient in the same prone position as in the passive technique and then apply one or more cups over the desired area of the posterior lower leg. With the cups in place, instruct the patient to dorsiflex and plantar flex the ankle to initiate an active cupping treatment (figure 6.14). This can also be performed in a standing position (figure 6.15).

Glide Technique over the Gastroc-Soleus Region

The glide techniques are best performed from the prone position. Make sure

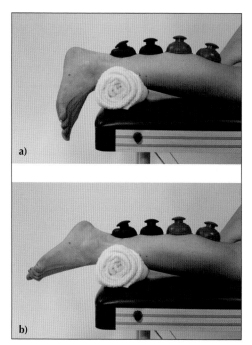

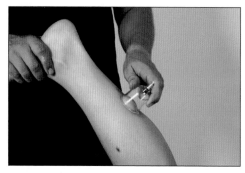

Figure 6.16. The glide technique for the gastroc-soleus region

Figure 6.14. Multiple cups on the posterior lower leg with (a) active dorsiflexion and (b) active plantar flexion

and alter the skin tension under the cup with a dorsiflexion motion. With the cup attached and leg suitably stabilized, glide the cup down the leg, up to but not over the back of the knee (figure 6.16). Repeat this process two or three times over the lower leg, monitoring for any significant reddening or pain provocation.

Passive, active, and glide calf muscle techniques

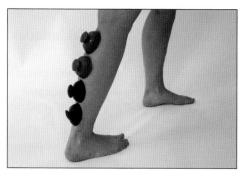

Figure 6.15. Active cupping with standing calf stretch

Cupping for Shin Pain

there is a liberal covering of wax, oil, or emollient over the posterior calf region. Apply one rigid cup just above the Achilles region, and then hold the foot with the other hand to both stabilize

Shin pain, or "shin splints," is usually caused by one of three common pathologies:

1. Anterior compartment syndrome, caused by overuse of the tibialis anterior muscle and swelling within the anterior fascial compartment.

2. Medial tibial stress syndrome (MTSS), caused by repetitive rapid-loading tasks like running and jumping.
3. Tibial stress fractures, also caused by repetitive rapid-loading tasks like running and jumping without enough time for bone remodeling.

Cupping should not be used over suspected fractures, which would include stress fractures, and therefore is not recommended for suspected tibial stress fractures. It is an option to use cupping to reduce the symptoms of MTSS, but I rarely use this technique myself. If you did want to try it, I would recommend using minimal vacuum because of the low amount of soft tissue in the area.

I have found the lateral shin application for anterior compartment syndrome useful and well received in practice.

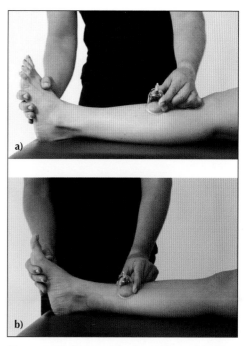

Figure 6.17. Using a single cup over (a) the lateral shin and (b) the medial shin, with the other hand stabilizing the lower leg

Passive Shin Techniques

With the patient seated, apply a cup to the medial or lateral shin and use the cup to mobilize the underlying soft tissue while stabilizing the leg with the other hand (figure 6.17).

Active Shin Techniques

With the patient seated so that the lower limb is non-weight bearing, apply one or more cups over the medial or lateral shin and then instruct the patient to dorsiflex

or plantar flex the ankle to begin the active cupping treatment (figure 6.18).

Glide-Cupping Techniques for the Shin

I find that the glide techniques work particularly well over the shin, with positive reports from patients. Glide cupping can be performed over the medial shin (figure 6.19) or over the lateral shin (figure 6.20). With both techniques, you will need to hold the ankle or foot to stabilize the lower leg.

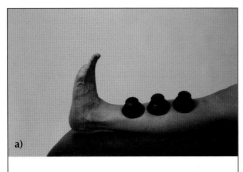

Passive, active, and glide shin techniques

Conclusion

While it can be occasionally difficult to get the cups to adhere to the foot and ankle, it is a very therapeutic intervention and one that some patients may be able to do for themselves if you wish to teach them some self-management strategies. This chapter has presented a broad range of techniques that can be used or adapted for many different pain presentations and rehabilitation requirements.

Figure 6.18. Cups over (a) the lateral shin and (b) the medial shin, with active plantar- and dorsiflexion

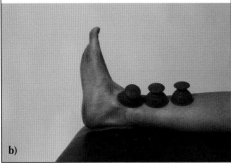

Figure 6.19 Medial shin glide cupping

References

Lopes, A. D., L. C. Hespanhol, S. S. Yeung, and L.O.P. Costa. 2012. "What are the main running-related musculoskeletal injuries? A systematic review." *Sports Medicine* 42(10): 891–905.

Thomas, M. J., R. Whittle, H. B. Menz, T. Rathod-Mistry, M. Marshall, and E. Roddy. 2019. "Plantar heel pain in middle-aged and older adults: Population prevalence, associations with health status and lifestyle factors, and frequency of healthcare use." *BMC Musculoskeletal Disorders* 20(1): 1–8.

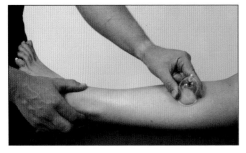

Figure 6.20. Lateral shin glide cupping

Cupping for the Knee and Thigh

How to Perform Cupping Techniques over the Knee and Thigh

Introduction

Knee pain can be caused by numerous different pathologies and is often diffuse in nature, spreading around the joint, making a specific diagnosis difficult. Younger patients often present with pain below the knee from Osgood-Schlatter's disease. Active adults commonly report a dull ache around the kneecap from a patellofemoral issue, and many older patients will have pain associated with osteoarthritis. Cupping can be used in the management of these conditions and many other pathologies around the knee.

Cupping can often be used directly over the knee, although this may not always be the best option. Cupping over the anterior thigh can often alleviate knee pain by generally reducing muscle tone and sensitivity over both the thigh and the knee. Cupping can also be used to target specific tender points over the

thigh that you find relate to the knee pain.

Most knee treatment plans include exercise rehabilitation, which is usually undertaken independently by the patient in the form of a prescribed home exercise plan. Despite the effectiveness of self-management programs, many patients continue to visit practitioners for passive treatment, advice, and symptomatic relief from symptom flare-ups. The use of cupping within such treatment sessions can be very helpful.

Getting Started

Using the standard application principles outlined in chapter 2, begin with the patient seated on a chair or treatment couch with the knee and thigh within easy reach to allow the mobilization of the cups.

Knee Techniques

Passive Knee-Cupping Techniques

The following passive technique is suitable for patients who require some symptomatic relief from knee pain and are not yet ready or willing to engage in more active methods. Place a cup on each side of the knee and mobilize them together (figure 7.1).

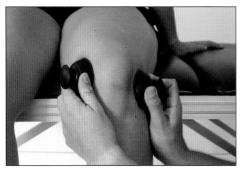

Figure 7.1. Passive knee technique with one cup on each side of the knee

Active Knee Cupping Techniques

The combination of cupping with non-weight-bearing knee bending, squatting, or lunge actions allows traditional cupping to fit in with a more movement-based approach to treatment. The following techniques should encourage the patient to move their knee. The introduction of a new sensory stimulus from the vacuum that then changes in its intensity when the skin is stretched and strained will hopefully feel therapeutic and promote movement.

Patients often describe a feeling of support around the joint during active cupping techniques. Figure 7.2 shows a non-weight-bearing application and figure 7.3 shows a weight-bearing slider lunge active-cupping drill.

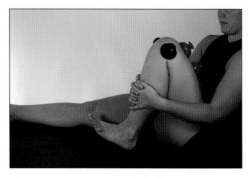

Figure 7.2. Cups around the knee and lower thigh with supine heel slides for knee flexion

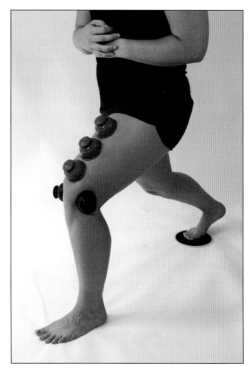

Figure 7.3. Cups placed as in figure 7.2 but with a lunge slide disc exercise

Glide Cupping Techniques for the Knee

The most effective glide technique to perform at the knee is the medial glide (figure 7.4). To perform the technique, I would recommend using minimal vacuum pressure and a liberal covering of emollient or similar. This is because the medial knee is not typically covered by much soft tissue or adipose tissue. Remember that you can always increase the vacuum pressure, but if you start with pressure that is too high and causes an intolerable amount of skin strain, it may dissuade your patient from any further cupping treatment. So always start with a low vacuum if you are unsure.

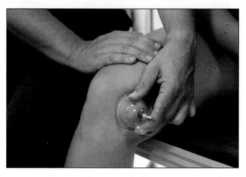

Figure 7.4. Single-cup glide cupping on the inner knee

Passive, active, and glide (seated and standing) for knee

Lateral Thigh Cupping Techniques

Receiving a vigorous massage over the lateral thigh, or iliotibial band (ITB), can often be an uncomfortable experience. Cupping offers a more comfortable method of soft-tissue mobilization thanks to the lifting effect of the vacuum. To perform a glide technique over the lateral thigh, I would recommend gliding down three different regions of the lateral leg: vastus lateralis, the ITB (figure 7.5), and the biceps femoris. Such an approach covers the lateral leg more fully than just navigating down the ITB in isolation. If your target is the ITB in relation to lateral leg pathologies, I would also recommend working on the glutes, as shown in chapter 8.

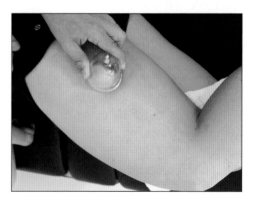

Figure 7.5. The ITB glide technique, side lying with pillow between knees

ITB glides

Hamstring Techniques

Hamstring strains are one of the most common sports injuries, and patients regularly present with self-reported tight hamstrings. As a result, the hamstrings are often a focus region during massage treatment and exercise rehabilitation. The simple but effective use of dry cupping for hamstring tension and pain is covered here.

Passive Hamstring Cupping Techniques

The passive treatment of the hamstrings using cupping is one of the easiest cupping treatment methods to perform. With the patient in prone, apply one cup over the back of the leg and mobilize the underlying soft tissue while using the other hand to stabilize the leg (figure 7.6). The cup can then be removed and placed on the next area of skin to be mobilized. It is typical to move along the length of the hamstrings by repeating this method up and down the leg following the application principles outlined in chapter 2.

An alternative position (figure 7.7) places the hamstrings into a lengthened, but not stretched, position, which may allow you to mobilize the upper hamstrings toward their ischial tuberosity origin.

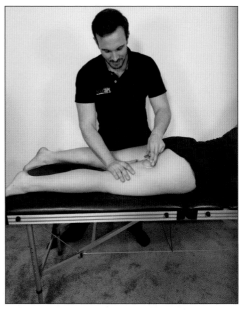

Figure 7.6. Prone hamstring cupping

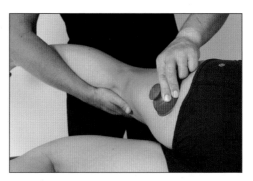

Figure 7.7. Side-lying hip-flexed passive hamstring cupping

Active Hamstring Cupping Techniques

The combination of cupping and active hamstring stretching is often described as feeling like a stretch and a massage

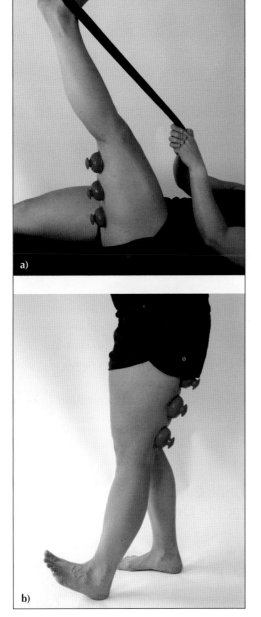

a)

b)

Figure 7.8. (a) Active hamstring cupping in supine with a leg straightener technique and (b) standing hamstring stretch

at the same time. Patients often enjoy the sensation of active hamstring cupping and as a result complete more repetitions during a given rehabilitation session. This is also a method that patients could do independently as part of a home routine. Apply a suitable number of cups to the posterior thigh, and then instruct the patient to engage in some active movement that lengthens the hamstrings (figure 7.8).

Glide Techniques for the Hamstrings

The therapeutic process of gliding the vacuum cups over the hamstrings is more easily achieved with a slight lengthening of the hamstrings to gently tighten the skin and create an easier gliding surface. You can then glide a cup up or down the leg (figure 7.9).

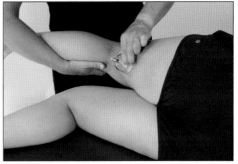

Figure 7.9. Side-lying hip-flexed hamstring glide cupping application

Passive, active, and glide for hamstrings

Quadriceps Techniques

As stated at the beginning of this chapter, soft-tissue mobilization, stretching, and strengthening exercises for the quadriceps often lead to both short-term and longer-term relief from knee pain. Cupping can be used to facilitate and enhance these treatment goals as well as provide treatment for more direct quadriceps issues like exercise-induced muscle soreness.

Passive Quadriceps Cupping Techniques

With the patient sitting comfortably, apply one or two cups over the thigh to mobilize the underlying soft tissue (figure 7.10).

Active Quadriceps Cupping Techniques

Apply the cups over the thigh and then instruct the patient to perform an active movement that lengthens and contracts the quadriceps. This could be achieved

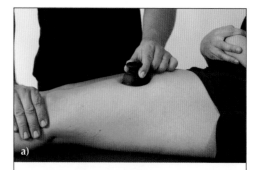

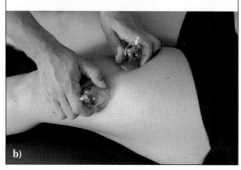

Figure 7.10. Passive quadriceps cupping with (a) one cup over the thigh and hand stabilizing the leg and (b) two cups over the thigh being mobilized by hand

in a non-weight-bearing position (figure 7.11) or a weight-bearing position (figure 7.12).

Glide Cupping Techniques for the Quadriceps

Apply one rigid cup over the thigh with the patient in a comfortable and stable resting position. As with all glide techniques, ensuring a degree of skin tension, but not necessarily stretch, will prevent the skin from puckering along the leading edge of the gliding cup (figure 7.13).

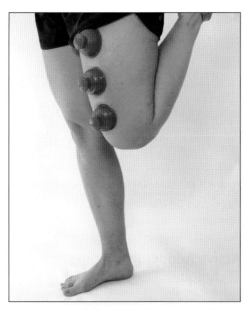

Figure 7.11. Cups over thigh, non-weight-bearing knee bend

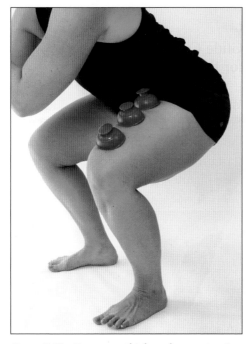

Figure 7.12. Cups over thigh and a squat action

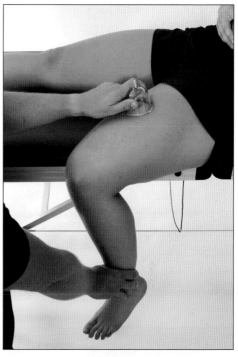

Figure 7.13. Patient long sitting supine with one thigh off the side of the couch so that knee flexion allows a tensioning over the anterior thigh

Passive, active, and glide for quadriceps

Adductor Techniques

Naturally, the inner thigh is a more neurologically sensitive and personally intimate part of the body in comparison to the lateral side of the leg. For this reason, some patients may not feel comfortable receiving cupping treatment to this area. If you do use cups over the inner thigh, I would suggest minimizing the vacuum in the first instance and following the adductor cupping guidelines outlined in this next section.

Passive Adductor Cupping Techniques

I find that one of the following positions is best for the passive application of the cups over the inner thigh (figure 7.14). Use one hand to stabilize the leg while you mobilize the cup and underlying soft tissue.

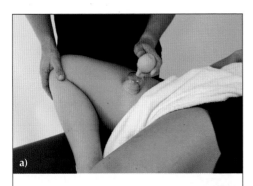
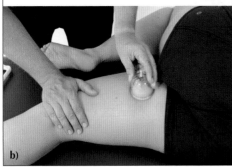

Figure 7.14. *Single cup over the inner thigh (a) in supine with hip flexed and abducted position and (b) side lying with hip flexed to allow access to the inner thigh of the lower leg*

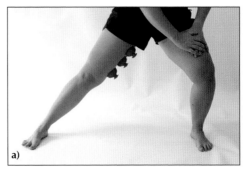

Figure 7.15. *Standing adductor stretch with three cups on the inner thigh*

Active Adductor Cupping Techniques

Apply one or more cups to the inner thigh and then instruct the patient to perform a suitable adductor stretch (figure 7.15).

Glide Cupping Techniques for the Adductors

With the patient in the passive adductor treatment position, glide a rigid cup over the adductor region. I recommend you start proximally and work toward the knee (figure 7.16).

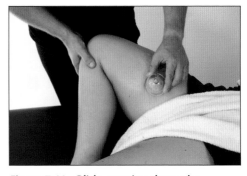

Figure 7.16. *Glide cupping down the adductor toward the knee*

Passive, active, and glide for adductors

choose to show people some cupping self-treatment regimes. Just remember to follow the general application principles outlined in chapter 2 and you should see some great results.

Conclusion

I hope you find the cupping techniques for the knee and thigh are well received by your patients. In some cases, you may

Cupping for Hip Pain

How to Use Vacuum-Cupping Techniques in the Management of Hip Pain

Introduction

Common causes of pain in the hip region include the following:

- Osteoarthritis
- Sciatic nerve irritation
- Piriformis syndrome
- Greater trochanteric pain syndrome
- Gluteal tendinopathy
- Femoroacetabular impingement
- Specific muscle- or tendon-related conditions.

This is by no means an exhaustive list, but represents the most common types of hip problem that cupping might be able to help manage as part of a modern treatment approach.

To claim that cupping can treat osteoarthritis would be spurious. It is more reasonable to suggest that cupping can be used to reduce the sensitivity of the soft tissue around the hip and offer a mechano-stimulus to support engagement in muscle-strengthening exercises, all as part of a holistic, person-centered, hip-osteoarthritis management plan.

The lateral hip and posterior gluteal muscle tissues are particularly responsive to soft-tissue mobilization.

The bony prominence of the greater trochanter can be an overly sensitive area when conditions such as greater trochanteric pain syndrome are present, but you may find that soft-tissue mobilization using a light vacuum offers a therapeutic intervention without causing further aggravation (figure 8.1).

The multilayered musculature of the gluteal region often responds well to massage, except in the case of peripheral nerve irritation of the sciatic nerve, where added pressure from manual

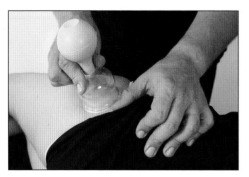

Figure 8.1. Example of a single cup over the lateral hip at the greater trochanter

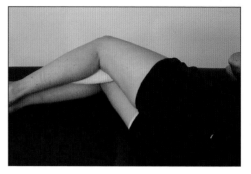

Figure 8.2. Side-lying position with a pillow between the knees

therapy may compound the problem. In such cases, the decompressive effect of cupping is especially helpful.

Caution: Hip Pain in Children

While hip pain is not an unusual presentation in the general population, hip pain in children is not normal and any child with hip pain should receive an urgent full medical examination with a low threshold for imaging investigation. For this reason, it would be sensible to consider undiagnosed hip pain in children as a contraindication for the use of cupping and other manual therapies.

Getting Started

Using the standard application principles outlined in chapter 2, begin with the patient in a side-lying position with the treatment hip uppermost and in slight flexion. Placing one or two pillows between the knees will stop lateral tension of the ITB over the lateral hip and make the treatment position more comfortable for the patient (figure 8.2).

Lateral and Posterior Hip Techniques

Passive Techniques

Secure a cup over the lateral or posterolateral hip (figure 8.3). Use one hand to mobilize the cup and underlying soft tissue while the other hand stabilizes the pelvis. These passive techniques can be performed in progressive ranges of hip flexion to offer a stretching stimulus to the hip musculature in combination with the passive soft-tissue mobilization.

Active Techniques

Place one or more cups over the posterolateral region of the hip and

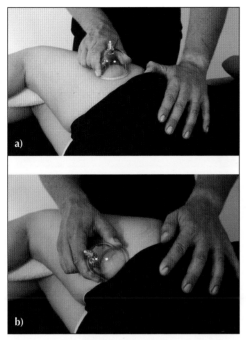

Figure 8.3. (a) Patient side lying, pillow between knees, single cup on lateral hip, and one hand stabilizing the pelvis; (b) cup more posterolateral

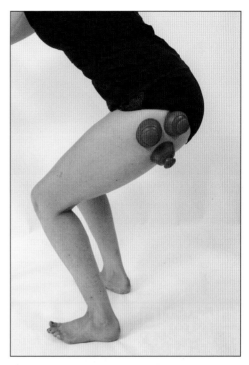

Figure 8.5. Cups on posterolateral region of the hip while patient performs an upper-body-assisted squat action

then instruct the patient to actively pull their hip into flexion (figure 8.4). You could also consider asking the patient

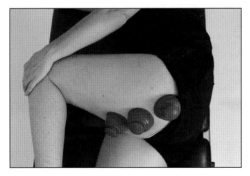

Figure 8.4. Cups on the posterolateral region of the hip, with patient side lying and pulling the hip into flexion

to perform a hip flexion action, like the squat, with the cups in place (figure 8.5). It is recommended that you use silicone cups because they will deform to prevent excessive vacuum and will not break if they become displaced during the active movements.

Glide Technique

Secure a rigid cup over the lateral hip with the patient in the side-lying position. Glide the cup slowly down from the lateral hip over the gluteal region (figure 8.6). Remove the cup and

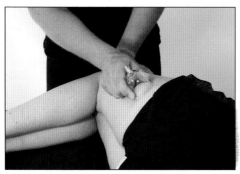

Figure 8.6. Gliding a cup slowly down from the lateral hip over the gluteal region

repeat the process, starting again from the lateral hip.

Passive, active, and glide for lateral hip and glutes

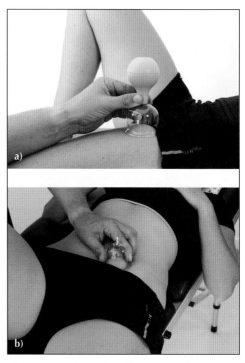

Figure 8.7. (a) Passive placement of one cup over upper thigh; (b) one cup over psoas

Anterior Hip Techniques

Cupping can be used over the anterior hip and thigh. One specific muscle that my students often ask about is the psoas (major and minor). Manual-therapy techniques commonly involve deep pressure down into the lateral abdomen, which clinicians often find is helpful but patients often report is painful or uncomfortable at best. I would encourage readers who perform psoas manual-therapy techniques to try utilizing cupping, with its unique ability to lift the soft tissue over the psoas.

Passive Techniques

With the patient in a comfortable supine position, apply one cup to the upper anterior thigh or over the anterior pelvis if you wish to target the psoas muscle. Use the cup to mobilize the underlying soft tissue, removing and repositioning as required (figure 8.7).

Active Techniques

Apply one or more cups over the anterior pelvis and thigh (figure 8.8a). Hip extension exercises can then be performed (figures 8.8b and c).

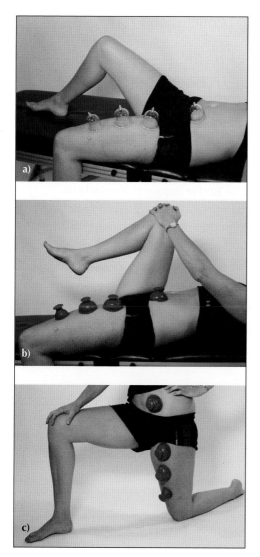

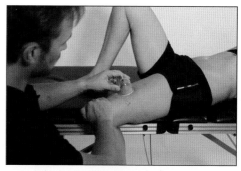

Figure 8.9. Glide cupping from a supine seated position with the leg off the side of the couch

with the treatment leg off the side of the couch to allow a lengthening of the rectus femoris and a slight extension of the hip joint (figure 8.9). The aim is to lengthen the soft tissue and not to create a stretching stimulus.

Passive, active, and glide for anterior hip

Figure 8.8. (a) Multiple cups placed over the anterior hip and thigh; (b) active cupping with supine hip extension off the side of the couch, other leg held up in flexion; (c) active cupping with kneeling hip extensor stretch

Glide Technique

The anterior hip glide technique is best performed in a supine seated position

Piriformis Technique

Piriformis syndrome is the term commonly used to describe the peripheral irritation of the sciatic nerve in the deep gluteal muscles, which include the piriformis muscle. I like to combine a hip stretch into flexion with cupping (figure 8.10). This provides a powerful combination of active tissue glide with passive mobilization.

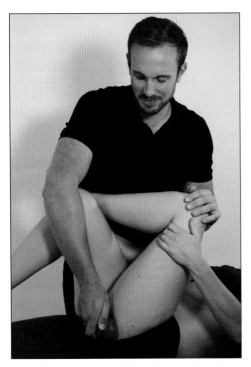

Figure 8.10. Supine piriformis stretch with single gluteal pod being mobilized

Conclusion

The negative pressure created by the cups provides an ideal tool to decompress the often-deep, multilayered soft tissue around the hip joint. It can be especially effective over the glutes when dealing with peripheral sciatic nerve irritation. Some therapists may also find it improves the patient's experience during psoas manual therapy. Experiment with the techniques shown in this chapter to find the best options for your patients.

Cupping for Back Pain

How to Use Vacuum-Cupping Techniques in the Management of Lower-Back Pain

Introduction

The incidence of lower-back pain varies within different societies and cultures around the world. For thousands of years, practitioners of different medical disciplines have attempted to treat back pain using different theories and methods. Massage, manipulation, acupuncture, and cupping have all received regular mention in historical medical texts. In the West, cupping became overshadowed by Western medicine and the rise of the evidence-based pharmaceutical industry. Vacuum cupping does not feature in any national back-pain guidelines either in the UK or USA and has until recently been overlooked by many physical therapists. In contrast, acupuncture, which could be considered a similar intervention with similar origins, has been widely integrated into Western pain management. I believe that cupping, when utilized correctly, may just require the opportunity to integrate with modern back-pain treatment approaches.

Placing a cup over the patient's perceived painful area provides a handle for mobilizing the soft tissue without the need to apply downward pressure, something that can be unduly painful in the case of lower-back pain. If you are fortunate enough to have received cupping therapy over your lower back, you will likely appreciate why it has become so popular. The feeling is so unique it is often said to be "indescribable," as it is not comparable to any other form of manual therapy.

Lower-back-pain treatment can be significantly aided with cupping, and so much more can be achieved beyond the traditional passive and static application methods. Cupping can transcend standard manual therapy and support the restoration of spinal movement and motor control. We will explore this further within this chapter.

Contraindications

While it is beyond the scope of this book to offer a full lumbar-spine assessment plan, this chapter does provide an opportunity to raise awareness of the spinal red flags, including cauda equina syndrome (CES).

CES is a rare but serious condition that if left untreated can lead to permanent loss of bladder and bowel control and sexual function. It is a condition that can be successfully treated if suspected and detected early. If your patient is experiencing any of the symptoms listed in box 1, instruct them to speak to a doctor or visit an emergency department on that same day. It is better to be overcautious if CES is suspected.

Box 1. Cauda Equina Syndrome Warning Signs

- Loss of feeling or pins and needles between the inner thighs or the groin
- Numbness around the genitals, buttocks, or anus
- Increased difficulty urinating, leaking, or loss of sensation
- Not knowing when your bladder is full or empty
- Loss of sensation in the genitals

If a patient reports any combination of the above, they should seek medical help immediately from a doctor or an emergency medical department.

Box 2. Serious Spinal Pathology Warning Signs

- History of trauma, including falls, collisions, and impacts
- Worsening pain that continues without movement and at rest
- History of cancer
- Known or suspected osteoporosis
- High temperature or feeling generally unwell

If a patient reports any of the above, they will need to be assessed by a medical professional before any treatment, including cupping, is considered.

Box 2 lists other signs of serious spinal pathology, which are therefore contraindications to treatment. Any patients suffering from or reporting any of these symptoms should report them to their doctor.

Stages of Nonspecific Back Pain

There are many causes of lower-back pain, and it remains a very unique experience for each individual.

This chapter will focus on techniques for nonspecific lower-back pain—this is the most common back-pain patient category. Patients with nonspecific lower-back pain have no history of spinal trauma and no symptoms of sciatic or other peripheral nerve involvement. The techniques will be most effective for acute back pain of less than six weeks duration but may also be utilized for more-persistent lower-back pain, while appreciating that longer-term back pain is often much more resistant to manual interventions.

Physiotherapist Dr. C. M. Norris (2020) described the back-pain recovery and rehabilitation process as passing through three distinct phases: reactive, recovery, and resilience. I am very much in favor of his approach.

When an episode of lower-back pain initially occurs, the patient is very reactive to the pain, often limiting movement and seeking to rest and immobilize as much as possible—this type of patient behavior is initially helpful to allow pain reduction and recovery. During this first phase, passive interventions, which could include cupping, are well received and appreciated by most patients. Once the patient feels the back pain has "settled," they should be guided to recover and restore normal spinal movement patterns. Cups can be used to augment the recovery phase, but not in the same manner they were used during the reactive phase. This is where we see the use of cups progressing from the constraints of traditional treatment to the innovative methods described later in this chapter.

The final phase, resilience, is the most exciting phase of rehabilitation. Sadly, it is one that is often ignored by bodyworkers and their patients, owing to the typically satisfactory reduction of pain and a lack of patient motivation to continue rehabilitation if no longer experiencing pain. In the resilience phase, as the name suggests, patients can build a resilience to the pain and dysfunction that come from the demands of normal daily life. This is often described as creating a functional buffer zone.

As mentioned previously, using cups for the treatment of lower-back pain requires a lot more than vacuuming the sore spots. The following treatment options are presented in a progressive order. You may be able to take a patient through the full regime in one session, or it may take multiple sessions to progress to the more advanced techniques.

Getting Started

Using the standard application principles outlined in chapter 2, begin with the patient in a resting position. This could be seated, prone lying, or side lying, depending on the patient's mobility and preference (figure 9.1).

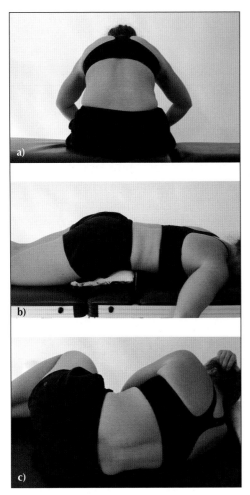

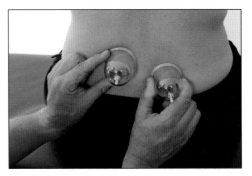

Figure 9.2. Seated cupping up the spine using two cups, one in each hand

with a low-to-moderate level of vacuum. This will allow the patient to familiarize themselves with the sensation, ask any questions regarding cupping, and begin to relax.

Following the introduction of one cup, the treatment can then progress by adding a second cup and mobilizing the soft tissue using the cups as handles, continuing this for 1 minute and then relocating the cups to avoid excessive skin marking (ecchymosis). Figure 9.2 shows an example of soft-tissue mobilization with two cups.

Figure 9.1. The three starting-position options: (a) seated, (b) prone lying, and (c) side lying

Active Cupping

Active cupping over the spine provides therapeutic movement in combination with the sensory stimulus of cupping. To achieve this, begin with the cups over the lower back, and then guide the patient to move through a specified

Passive Cupping

The starting position should be as comfortable as possible for the patient before the cups are applied. You may wish to start with just one cup applied

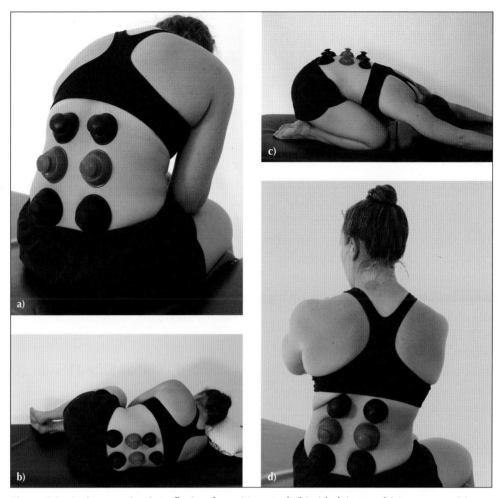

Figure 9.3. Active cupping into flexion from (a) seated, (b) side lying, and (c) prone position, plus (d) seated rotation

range of motion. Figure 9.3 provides examples of active flexion (figure 9.3a–c) and rotation (figure 9.3d) progressions. Large ranges of motion can lead to a loss of vacuum as the skin movement breaks the seal around the cup. For this reason, make sure you are not using glass or other breakable cups.

Advanced Techniques

Active cupping techniques can be enhanced with passive soft-tissue mobilization to create an enhanced tissue shear during an identified movement restriction. The tissue shear can be applied to either assist or resist the movement or may alternate between the two. Advanced technique examples for spinal rotation, lumbar flexion, and side flexion are shown below.

Advanced Lumbar Rotation Technique

Begin with the patient seated, with their back accessible. Assess the direction of rotation restriction—i.e., right or left. Then place two cups on or just above the glutes on the same side as the rotation restriction, at an oblique angle (figure 9.4a). The aim is to place the cups along one of the myofascial lines that run across the spine. The cups can then be gently mobilized in the opposite direction to the active rotation to create tissue resistance and a tolerable level of shear strain (figure 9.4b).

An alternative method would be to assist the soft-tissue glide by mobilizing the cups in the same direction as the rotation (figure 9.4c). Following three or four end-range rotations coupled with the assisted or resisted soft-tissue mobilization, the patient should experience less resistance into rotation. If required, the treatment can be repeated and the cups can be reapplied further up the myofascial line (figure 9.4d).

Advanced Lumbar Flexion Technique

Begin with the patient seated, with the feet raised to flex the hips. The patient should then bend forward into pain-free lumbar flexion (figure 9.5a). Apply two cups over the paraspinal muscles at the level of the upper lumbar spine. Apply a shearing force through the cups by resisting the forward flexion with a downward counter-tension by pulling the cups gently downward (figure 9.5b). Repeat this maneuver as the cups are relocated at intervals down the lumbar spine and over the upper sacroiliac-joint region (SIJ) (figure 9.5d).

Advanced Lumbar Side-Flexion Technique

Begin with the patient in a neutral sitting position with approximately 90 degrees of flexion at the hips. Place one large cup over the region of the quadratus lumborum on the side you wish to stretch. Instruct the patient to reach up above their head and side flex in the opposite direction, while opposing the side flexion with downward counter-pressure using the cup (figure 9.6). Repeat this maneuver three to four times before retesting the patient's side flexion.

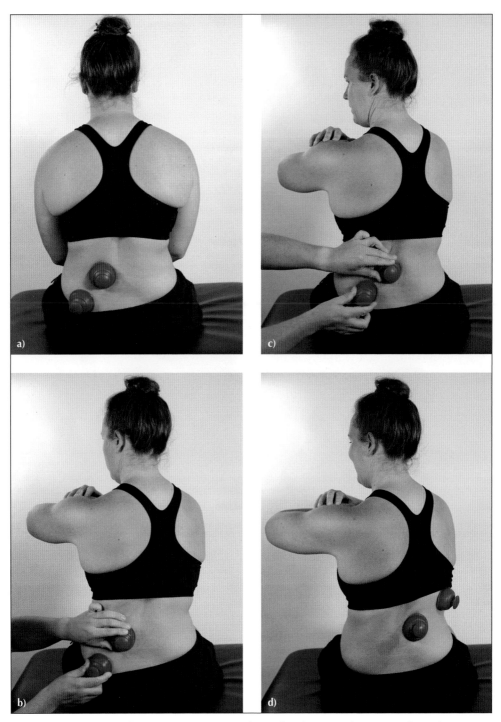

Figure 9.4. (a) Start with two cups on or just above the glutes on the same side as the rotation restriction at an oblique angle; (b) mobilize in the opposite direction or (c) in the same direction; (d) cups can be reapplied further up the myofascial line

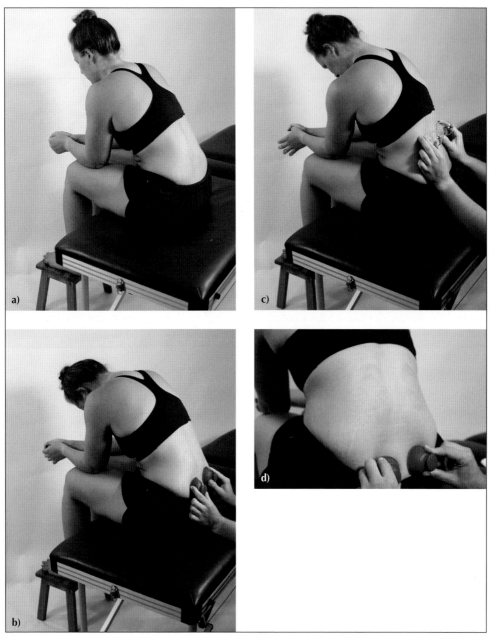

Figure 9.5. (a) Patient seated with feet raised to create a squat position and then flexed forward; (b) two cups over the paraspinal muscles with a shearing force to resist the forward flexion by pulling the cups gently downward; (c) example using rigid plastic cups; (d) pods over the SIJ region

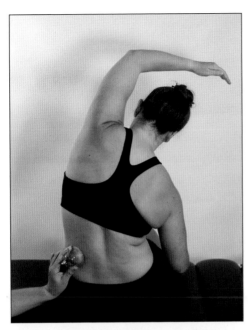

Figure 9.6. With one large cup over the quadratus lumborum, the patient reaches up and side flexes in the opposite direction, while you oppose the side flexion with downward pressure through the cup

Bringing It All Together

Once a patient becomes familiar with cupping therapy and regains confidence in their spinal motion, then the methods presented in this chapter can be delivered progressively during a single treatment session, with some potential customization to suit individual patients.

Figure 9.7 shows a series of photographs taken during a progressive lumbar-spine cupping treatment. You will note

that figure 9.7d shows the use of a deep squat to achieve the full range of lumbar flexion.

Cupping for Back-Pain Rehabilitation

The sensory experience of vacuum cupping can offer more than just a pleasant sensation. The lumbar spine is a region that lacks the ability to calibrate its movement with simple visual feedback.* As a result, educating back-pain patients in the performance of restorative movement patterns can be challenging. Movement performance can be enhanced with increased sensory input, and this is often achieved with careful hand placement, also known as tactile facilitation, but it can also be achieved with vacuum cups, which have the advantage of being able to cover a larger area and provide a more intense and novel sensory input when compared with the touch of a hand.

For example, if you are teaching a patient to flex the lumbar spine, they may struggle to feel whether the spine is indeed flexing. However, with strategically placed cups (figure 9.8), an

---

* Without the use of mirrors or cameras, it is not possible to witness the movement of some parts of the body, including the lumbar spine and shoulder blades. When you cannot see the movement, it makes it difficult to assess the success or failure of any given movement pattern, and therefore difficult to correct it.

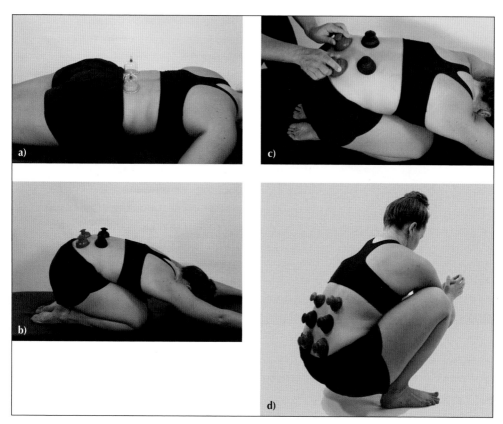

Figure 9.7. (a) Passive lumbar cupping (two cups) in prone position; (b) Balasana *yoga stretch (four pods); (c)* Balasana *plus shearing; (d) deep squat (six pods)*

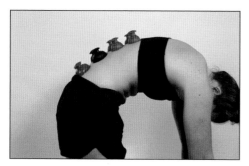

Figure 9.8. Eight cups plus four-point kneeling with active spinal flexion and extension

intense stretching under the cups will be felt on flexion of the lumbar spine, which will provide the feedback and sensory reference to perform the flexion action correctly and to learn a new movement pattern.

Lumbar techniques

Conclusion

The many different ways in which cupping can be incorporated into lower-back pain management highlights how versatile this treatment modality has the potential to be. You may wish to follow the guidance set out in this chapter or use the concepts to improve your current approaches to back pain. Whichever route you decide to take, the intention of this chapter was to present a modern methodology that allows practitioners to break away from the limitations of traditional cupping and begin an integration with the modern evidence-based approaches to back pain.

References

Myers, T. W. 2013. *Anatomy Trains E-Book: Myofascial Meridians for Manual and Movement Therapists.* Elsevier Health Sciences.

Norris, C. M. 2020. "Back rehabilitation: The 3R's approach." *Journal of Bodywork and Movement Therapies* 24(1): 289–99.

Cupping for Shoulder Pain

Cupping Techniques to Help Manage Shoulder Pain and Enhance Rehabilitation from Injury

Introduction

During normal daily tasks the shoulder joint serves the upper limb by positioning the arm and hand to allow the control and manipulation of objects, such as lifting a hot cup of coffee, turning the steering wheel of your car, or retrieving something from your back pocket. For this reason, shoulder pain can have a significant impact on normal daily life and be very distressing.

Shoulder pain can be caused by many different conditions of the joint, and the true cause of most shoulder pain often remains in question. It is often helpful to divide shoulder pain into three broad categories so that the most suitable treatment approach can be utilized:

- The painful shoulder
- The stiff shoulder
- The hypermobile shoulder.

The Painful Shoulder

Shoulder pain syndrome is a term which describes a shoulder that is painful but with a near-normal range of passive motion. The patient often displays a reduced active range of motion because of the pain, but when the therapist moves the patient's shoulder passively, there is a notable increased range of motion, indicating the restriction is caused by pain rather than a physical joint restriction. Other terms for this type of shoulder problem include subacromial impingement and rotator cuff tendinopathy.

The Stiff Shoulder

A stiff shoulder will have a limited range of motion both actively and passively. The joint restriction will have a physical feel to it, with or without the presence of pain. Many things can cause a shoulder to become stiff.

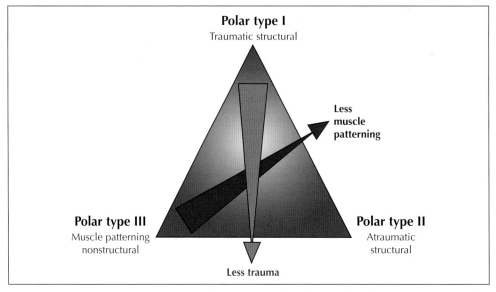

Figure 10.1. The Bayley triangle shows the Stanmore classification for glenohumeral instability

Perhaps the best known is frozen shoulder, also known as adhesive capsulitis but more recently termed shoulder contracture syndrome. It's hard to keep up with all of these terminology changes! Shoulder stiffness may also follow surgery (including mastectomy) and fracture, commonly humeral spiral fracture. Osteoarthritis of the glenohumeral joint is another potential cause of a stiff shoulder.

The Hypermobile Shoulder

Occasionally patients will present with shoulder pain and an above average range of motion. There are three potential causes of excessive mobility at the shoulder, with typical overlap between the three causes. These are shown in the Bayley triangle (figure 10.1).

Contraindications

Patients experiencing shoulder pain after direct trauma or those reporting continual pain, even at rest, should be assessed by a medical professional. They would not be suitable for manual therapy, including the treatments outlined in this chapter.

Getting Started

My students are often surprised by the multiple ways cups can be used around the shoulder to help reduce pain and to augment exercise rehabilitation. I will explain and demonstrate the most effective shoulder applications in this chapter.

Using the standard application principles outlined in chapter 2, begin with the patient in a resting position. This could be seated or side lying (figure 10.2).

The starting position should be as comfortable as possible for the patient before the cups are applied. You may wish to start with just one cup applied with a low-to-moderate level of vacuum. This will allow the patient to become familiar with the sensation and begin to relax. When manually mobilizing a fixed cup on the shoulder in a seated position, I recommend using one hand to mobilize the cup and the other to stabilize over the shoulder. The single cup can be mobilized in a circular motion to the point of tissue resistance, which

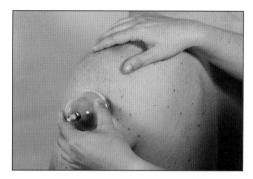

Figure 10.3. Cupping over the deltoid using a single cup with one hand stabilizing

provides the feeling of a deep and relieving massage over the deltoid region (figure 10.3).

Active Cupping for the Glenohumeral Joint

The therapeutic benefits of cupping can combine with the therapeutic benefits of movement to produce a more involved treatment process. The best way to perform an active cupping technique over the deltoid region is shown in figure 10.4a. Depending on the size of your patient and the size of the cups you are using, aim to locate four cups around the shoulder. The patient should then be encouraged to move the shoulder in different directions to feel a stretch and shearing sensation created by the vacuum within the cups (figure 10.4b).

For the more apprehensive patient who requires a more-passive, guided approach, I would recommend the side-lying technique shown in figure 10.4c.

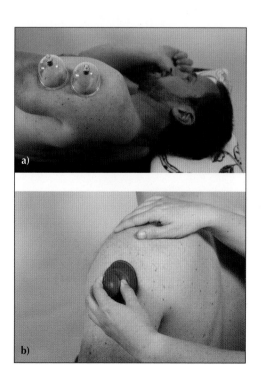

Figure 10.2. Starting position for shoulder cupping: (a) side lying; (b) seated

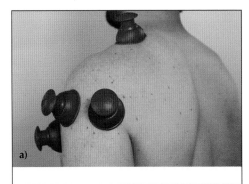

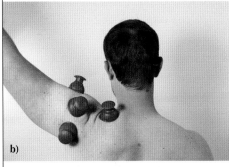

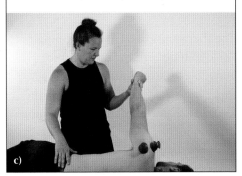

Figure 10.4. (a) Location of the four pods over the three deltoids and one over the upper traps; (b) pods in situ with patient moving the arm, showing abduction/ adduction; (c) patient side lying with pods in situ and therapist moving patient's arm

Glide Cupping

Gliding the cups up from the lateral arm and over the deltoid pulls and mobilizes the skin and muscle in a way that is often described as relieving and relaxing by patients. This is a very passive approach to the treatment of shoulder pain, but one that will most likely offer symptomatic relief and allow more confidence to get the joint moving again.

To perform this style of glide cupping over the lateral arm, you will need rigid cups and a layer of emollient spread liberally over the lateral and upper arm to cover the treatment area. Begin with the patient seated below you, so that you can pull the cups upward rather than need to push them (figure 10.5a). Once they reach the top of the arm, the cups should come away from the skin as the contour of the shoulder breaks the seal and releases the vacuum (figure 10.5b).

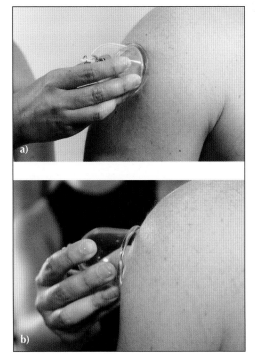

Figure 10.5. (a) Glide cupping up over the deltoid with the patient seated; (b) release of the cup as it comes up over the shoulder

Passive, active, and glide for GHJ

Scapular Cupping Techniques

Many patients report tender points in the muscles around the scapula. These are often described as knots or referred to as trigger points. Separate from the academic discussions surrounding the relevance of these sore spots and the efficacy of various treatment approaches, the clinical use of manual therapy for these tender points remains a common and well-received intervention. Techniques include direct pressure, acupuncture, and vibration. We can also use the focal nature of the vacuum to alter tissue tension and desensitize the nervous system.

The simple but effective techniques shown here rely on the correct placement of the cups over the patient-reported sore spots (figure 10.6). Once in place, the cup or cups can be mobilized and gently lifted from their fixed position to provide a deeper stimulus.

Top Tip

When we discussed the biomechanics of cupping in chapter 3, it was noted that the rim of the cup compresses into the skin. For this reason, it is helpful to use as large a cup as possible, with the tender spot centralized within the cup.

Active Cupping for the Scapulothoracic Joint

Stiffness and poor movement control of the scapulothoracic joint is common in the general population. People with shoulder pain often benefit from any treatments and exercises that get the shoulder blades and thoracic spine moving to the best of their ability. This next technique is one of my favorite cupping applications for promoting movement around the shoulder girdle and thoracic spine.

To perform the technique, apply cups over the upper back (figure 10.7a). The cups should be applied with the patient in a neutral position, such as sitting or prone lying. Once the cups are in place, the patient should be instructed to fully stretch forward to protract the scapula and flex the thoracic spine (figure 10.7b). This should then

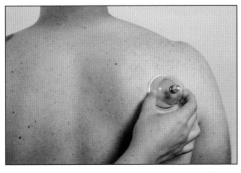

Figure 10.6. Cupping placement around the scapula, using one cup over infraspinatus

be followed by a controlled move to the opposite position of thoracic extension and scapular retraction (figure 10.7c), repeated a few times.

In addition to the benefits of stretching and mobilizing the shoulder girdle, the extra stimulus from the cups offers an increased sensory input that may serve to improve proprioception and motor control of this region with potentially positive benefits to shoulder function.

Glide Cupping the Thoracic Spine

The combination of a manual glide with inverted pressure down over the thoracic erector spinae muscles provides the patient with a satisfying and unique treatment experience. The technique can be performed entirely passively or with a little bit of active motion. Rigid cups will work best for this technique, and the treatment area should be lubricated to allow the smooth flow of the cups over the skin.

Begin with the patient lying in prone (figure 10.8a) or in a seated position with the feet on a secure surface (figure 10.8b). I find this technique is best performed down over the upper back rather than up, as this helps the cups flow over the skin in a smoother fashion. The seated technique can incorporate some active flexion as the cups are slid down the upper back (figure 10.8c).

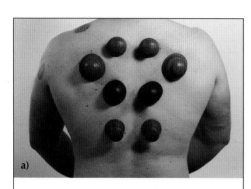
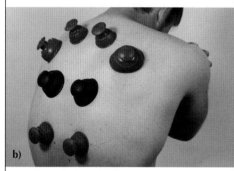
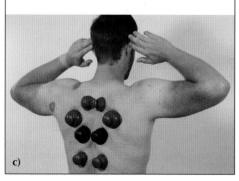

Figure 10.7. (a) Cup placement for scapulothoracic-joint active cupping; (b) full stretch forward to protract scapula and flex thoracic spine; (c) thoracic extension and scapular retraction

Passive, active, and glide for scapula

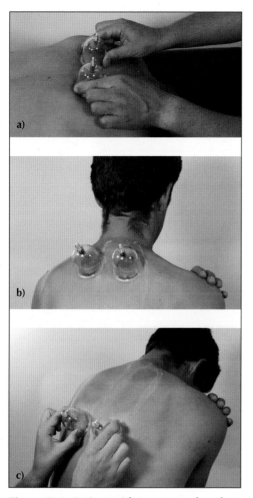

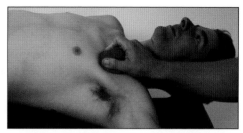

Figure 10.9. Patient supine with arm off the side of the couch, but held by the therapist, and one cup placed over the upper chest

to cup the pectoralis minor through the armpit is contraindicated.

The technique I recommend is a shearing method over the upper chest using one cup placed over the mid-portion of the pectoralis major region. The cup can then be mobilized toward the midline and the arm gently stretched back into extension (figure 10.9).

 **Shearing for pecs**

Figure 10.8. Patient with two cups placed at the base of the neck, (a) prone and (b) seated with feet on a stool; (c) active flexion cupping technique

Shearing Technique for the Pectoralis Major

Many of my students are keen to learn cupping methods for "tight pecs"—remember: we cannot use cups in the axilla because of the lymph node cluster and other patient comfort considerations, and therefore attempting

Shearing Technique for the Latissimus Dorsi and Teres Major

This next technique is helpful for those with stiff shoulders who struggle to achieve full abduction and those suffering from training-related muscle tension in the latissimus dorsi muscles. To perform the technique, start with the patient

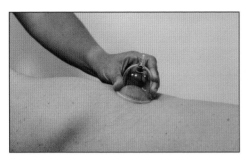

Figure 10.10. Side-lying latissimus dorsi shearing technique

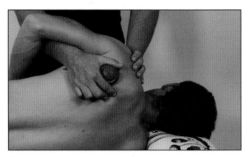

Figure 10.11. Patient side lying for scapular mobilization

side lying and passively abduct the arm toward the end of the available range. Secure one cup just below the posterior part of the axilla, and then use the cup to mobilize the soft tissue inferiorly while moving the arm superiorly to create the shearing effect (figure 10.10).

Note: This technique is not advised if the initial positioning causes significant pain for the patient.

possible to grip the scapula, then a large cup with a moderate level of vacuum can provide a suitable scapular handle for mobilization.

Scapular mobilization

Shearing for lats

Conclusion

This chapter has demonstrated how the versatility of cupping can be used to help manage shoulder dysfunction from a variety of causes. The different methods of cupping around the shoulder offer much more than passive pain relief. The combination of movement and improved proprioception significantly enhances the treatment effect. As with all methods, patients may benefit initially from simple techniques before being taught more-advanced applications that require a careful interplay between the therapist and patient.

Advanced Scapular Technique

With the patient lying on their side, it is usually possible to passively mobilize the scapula by gripping under its medial border to create a scapular lift (figure 10.11). With some patients, this may not be possible because of a lack of mobility or pain guarding. If it is not

Cupping for Wrist, Hand, and Elbow Pain

How to Use Vacuum-Cupping Techniques in the Management of Wrist, Hand, and Elbow Pain

Introduction

The repetitious use of our hands and wrists during modern life leaves them susceptible to repetitive strain injuries (RSIs). While the predicted epidemic of "texter's thumb" from the pre-smartphone era never materialized, and gadgets and workstations have ergonomically improved, as have health and safety policies, office and manual workers continue to frequently report hand, wrist, and elbow pain. It is interesting to note that both office workers and manual workers are at high risk of upper-limb RSIs, even though there are clear differences in the load and intensity of their working activities. RSIs continue to have a significant economic burden on society because of time off work; in relation to this, they can necessitate changes of career and affect quality of life.

While RSI is the most common cause of upper-limb pain, it is by no means the only one. Injury can occur from trauma or the pain may be caused by more gradual degenerative disorders.

The vacuum created by cupping can be used to mobilize and massage the soft tissue around the hand and wrist, as well as around the forearm and up to the elbow. In some cases, you may also consider educating the patient to perform the cupping techniques as a self-treatment. Traditional cupping methods would preclude the option for patient-led self-cupping owing to safety and practical difficulties, but the modern approach to cupping presented in this book, combined with modern, easy-to-use cups, provides new possibilities for safe and effective self-cupping.

Lateral Forearm Techniques

Cupping over the lateral forearm can provide symptomatic relief from lateral epicondylalgia—also known as "tennis elbow"—by desensitizing the teno-osseous region over the lateral epicondyle and reducing tension in the wrist extensor muscles by massaging the forearm musculature.

Passive or Self-Application Lateral Elbow Techniques

To perform a passive technique here, place one cup over the lateral elbow using the application principles outlined in chapter 2. With the cup secured in place, move it to mobilize the skin and soft tissue beneath (figure 11.1). Cupping further down the forearm over the wrist extensors can also provide therapeutic relief (figure 11.2).

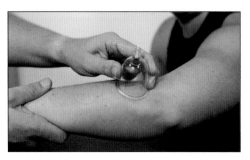

Figure 11.2. Single cup placed over the lateral forearm with forearm resting on table

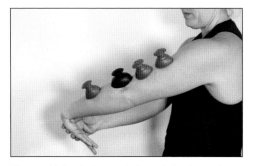

Figure 11.3. Active cupping of the lateral forearm, with tennis-elbow stretch demonstrated

Glide Cupping over the Lateral Forearm

Apply a liberal covering of wax or oil before securing a rigid cup over the lateral elbow with a moderate vacuum. Stabilize the arm with one hand, or if self-applied, rest the arm on a table to stabilize it while gliding the cup around the lateral elbow and down the forearm (figure 11.4).

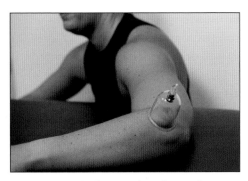

Figure 11.1. Single cup placed over the lateral elbow with forearm resting on table

Active Cupping over the Lateral Forearm

Place cups over the lateral forearm and elbow and over the lateral upper arm. With the cups secured in place, instruct the patient to perform wrist-extensor stretching exercises (figure 11.3).

Passive, active, and glide for lateral elbow

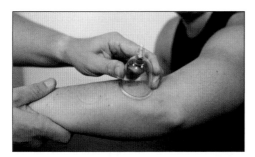

Figure 11.4. Single cup for glide cupping around the lateral elbow

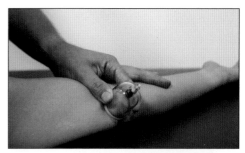

Figure 11.5. Single cup over the medial elbow

Medial Forearm Techniques

Cupping over the medial forearm can provide symptomatic relief from medial epicondylalgia by desensitizing the teno-osseous region over the medial epicondyle and reducing wrist-flexor muscle tension by massaging the medial forearm musculature.

Passive or Self-Application Techniques

Cupping can be used to mobilize the musculature of the medial forearm from the wrist to the medial elbow (figure 11.5). Be aware of the superficial location of the ulnar nerve over the inner elbow, and avoid creating a vacuum directly over this location (figure 11.6).

Active Cupping Technique

To perform an active cupping technique for medial-elbow pain, begin by securing one or more cups over the medial elbow and forearm and then

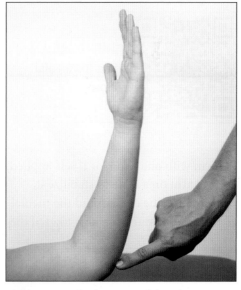

Figure 11.6. The location of the ulnar nerve at the elbow

instruct the patient to stretch the wrist flexors (figure 11.7).

Glide Cupping over the Medial Forearm

Apply a liberal covering of wax or oil over the medial forearm and elbow and then secure a rigid cup over the medial elbow with a moderate vacuum. Stabilize

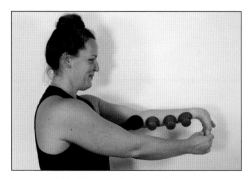

Figure 11.7. Medial elbow and forearm active cupping

Passive, active, and glide for medial elbow

the arm with one hand, or if self-applied, rest the arm on a table to stabilize it, while gliding the cup around the medial elbow and down the forearm toward the wrist (figure 11.8).

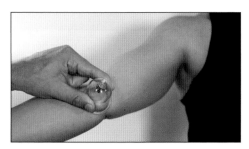

Figure 11.8. Medial-elbow glide cupping

Carpal Tunnel Cupping

Passive, active, and glide cupping can be performed over the carpal tunnel and up into the forearm. A passive application

can be performed by placing the cup directly over the carpal tunnel with a low-to-moderate level of vacuum. You may find that a softer silicone cup will more readily form a vacuum over the wrist. The cup can then be mobilized in accordance with the standard application principles (figure 11.9). Active cupping can be performed with the simple addition of wrist flexion and extension (figure 11.10).

Glide cupping can also be performed (figure 11.11); this was the technique of choice in a study by Mohammadi

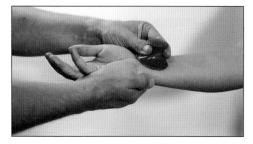

Figure 11.9. A single cup being mobilized over the carpal tunnel

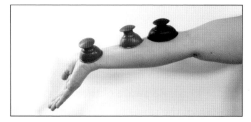

Figure 11.10. Cups over the carpal tunnel and forearm with wrist extension

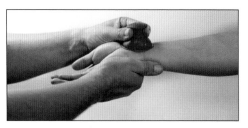

Figure 11.11. Carpal-tunnel glide cupping

Research Focus

A 2019 trial published in the *Physiotherapy Research International* journal by Mohammadi et al. reported on the results of incorporating cupping into the management of carpal tunnel syndrome using a randomized controlled trial design. The authors studied fifty-six patients, who all received transcutaneous electrical nerve stimulation and ultrasound. Half of the group—twenty-eight patients—also received ten sessions of cupping over the dorsum of the wrist, over and above the carpal tunnel using a 4-minute glide-cupping application. It is also interesting to note the additional use of a silicone interface around the base of the cup to maintain a vacuum over the contours of the wrist. In clinic this can be achieved by using a softer silicone cup.

The study measured symptom severity, functional status, distal sensory latency, and distal motor latency, reporting greater improvements for all measures (except the distal motor latency) in the group receiving cupping. The main theorized mechanism of action was the biomechanical pull on the transverse carpal ligament, which may improve the intra-neuronal blood flow to the median nerve as it passes through the carpal tunnel.

The authors did identify some of the study's limitations—the lack of previous studies for comparison and the low level of vacuum used as standard for each patient, suggesting that higher levels of vacuum may have resulted in improved treatment outcomes in some patients, possibly dependent on initial symptom severity.

Carpal Tunnel Syndrome

Carpal tunnel syndrome is the most common peripheral-nerve entrapment pathology (figure 11.12). The condition is caused by irritation of the median nerve as it passes through the carpal tunnel on the palmar side of the wrist. The median nerve's normal motion and fluid flow can be affected by swelling, bony changes, or ligamentous changes within the carpal tunnel.

A compromised median nerve will produce sensory loss in the hand and loss of muscle function. Reports of

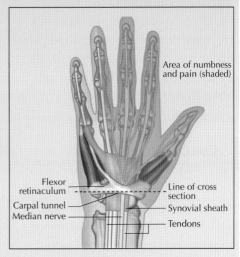

Figure 11.12. Carpal tunnel syndrome

Carpal Tunnel Syndrome (Continued)

a numb and weak hand are typical. Nerve conduction tests pass an electrical stimulus through the nerve to measure the delay, also known as the latency, in the signal. The results are separated into distal sensory latency and distal motor latency. The sensory latency is more sensitive to early changes in nerve function.

The nerve testing is often referred to as antidromic, which means that the nerve impulse is sent in reverse to perform the test and record the speed of the impulse transfer.

and colleagues (2009)—see the research focus box for more details.

Active, passive, and glide for carpal tunnel

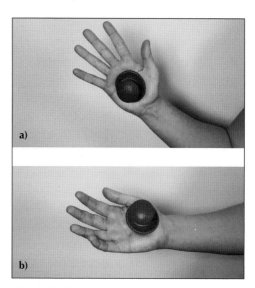

a)

b)

Figure 11.13. (a) Cupping of the palm of the hand and (b) of the thumb

Cupping the Hand

Cupping in the palm of the hand or over the base of the thumb may offer symptomatic relief from localized pain and tension and provide a therapeutic self-treatment option. Examples are shown in figure 11.13.

patients some self-cupping techniques for ongoing relief.

Conclusion

Cupping can provide rapid relief from pain and tension at the elbow, wrist, or hand. Many pathologies of these joints are persistent in nature, and I would therefore encourage you to teach your

Reference

Mohammadi, S., M. M. Roostayi, S. S. Naimi, and A. A. Baghban. 2019. "The effects of cupping therapy as a new approach in the physiotherapeutic management of carpal tunnel syndrome." *Physiotherapy Research International* 24(3): e1770.

Cupping for Neck Pain

How to Use Vacuum-Cupping Techniques in the Management of Neck Pain

Introduction

Neck pain is a common affliction for people throughout the world and is reported more frequently in higher-income countries and among office and computer workers (Hoy et al. 2010). New episodes of neck pain will often resolve spontaneously, but around 50 percent of neck-pain sufferers will continue to experience pain or have regular reoccurrences (Cohen 2015). This leads to frequent health-care visits for pain relief and advice.

Neck pain is rarely a simple physical problem, and a successful recovery is often influenced by the broader determinants of health (Côté et al. 2003). Many patients report that their neck pain gets worse with increased stress, and it is postulated that psychological factors may be more influential on recovery from an acute bout of nontraumatic neck pain than physical factors (Wirth et al. 2016).

Despite the need to assess and treat the neck with nonphysical strategies to manage the multifaceted causes, patients often expect and look forward to some manual therapy and pain relief during a treatment session. Even if the relief is initially short-lived, meeting a patient's expectations with a therapeutic intervention will often help to build the patient's trust and confidence in the longer-term self-management strategies that you may wish to suggest.

In this chapter I will show you some cupping techniques for neck pain, which begin with simple passive applications and progress to include active neck movements and more advanced options. The techniques have been tried and tested successfully on my patients, and I hope you will find them equally successful with your own patients. There are also studies that support the use of traditional cupping for the management of neck pain (Chi et al. 2016; Lauche et al. 2012).

Before we begin, this chapter aims to show you how to use dry cupping safely and effectively on the neck. It does not include a guide to neck assessment, but I would like to take this opportunity to list a few neck-pain symptoms that would indicate the need for an immediate medical referral and be a contraindication to treatment. These are often referred to as "red flags" in health care.

Cervical Red Flags during Assessment

- New sudden severe headache
- Dizziness
- Visual disturbance
- Slurred speech
- Facial muscle weakness
- Facial sensation loss
- Drooping eyelid

Patients who demonstrate or report these signs should not receive any treatment and should receive immediate medical attention.

Separate from the listed cervical red flags, my YouTube channel—"The Physio Channel"—contains a neck-assessment playlist that you may find helpful.

Getting Started

Using the standard application principles outlined in chapter 2, begin with the patient in a resting position.

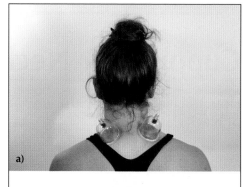
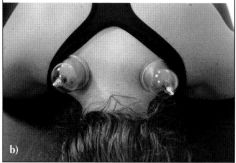

Figure 12.1. The starting-position options for neck-pain cupping: (a) seated or (b) prone lying, with cups in situ

This could be seated or prone lying (figure 12.1). I prefer performing cupping for the neck with the patient in a seated position because it is easier to move the head around passively and actively. I have included the prone option as an alternative.

Passive Cupping Techniques for the Neck

The starting position should be as comfortable as possible for the patient before the cups are applied. You may wish to start with just one cup, applied with a low-to-moderate level of vacuum. This will allow the patient to familiarize themselves with the sensation and begin to relax. When manually mobilizing a fixed cup on the neck in a seated position, I recommend using one hand to mobilize the cup and keeping the other hand free to support or guide the movement of the head. If the patient's torso is moving around too much because of the force of the cup mobilization, then you may need to apply the technique in the prone position to stabilize the torso.

You may find it advantageous to work with two cups, beginning from the lower trapezius region and then removing and relocating in stages up to the base of the neck and out over the shoulders (figure 12.2).

Top Tip

From experience, I have found that cupping around the neck and shoulders causes a faster reddening (ecchymosis) response. Patients have little desire to have red circles showing on their neck for fear people will assume they were caused by a romantic encounter (hickeys!) and not therapeutic cupping. To lessen the ecchymosis, I usually reduce each vacuum to 30 seconds or less before relocating the cups. I am also extra careful not to apply too much vacuum.

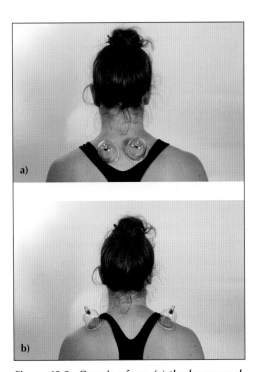

Figure 12.2. Cupping from (a) the lower neck and then (b) out over the upper trapezius

Active Movement

Because the neck is such a mobile part of our body, the combination of cupping with active movement creates a profound combination of stretching and massage. This treatment strategy often encourages patients to move their head around to experience the therapeutic pulling and shearing of the vacuum. This style of application typically utilizes four or more cups placed over the lower neck, upper back, and upper shoulders (figure 12.3).

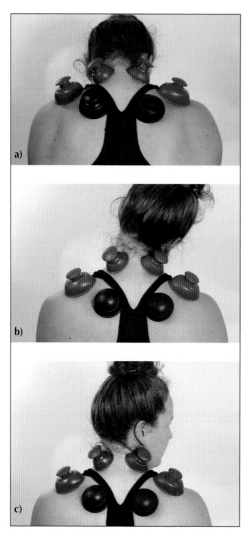

Figure 12.3. Cupping the lower neck and upper shoulders with (a) flexion, (b) side flexion, and (c) rotation

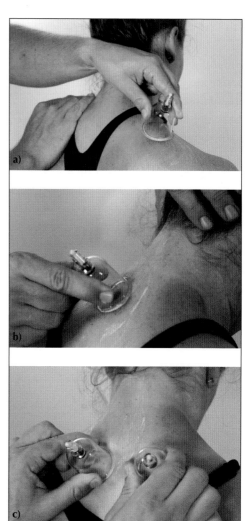

Figure 12.4. Glide cupping for the neck: (a) from the neck out over the upper traps; (b) from the neck down over the upper back; (c) using two cups with movement

Glide Cupping

Glide cupping can then be applied, while encouraging the patient to side flex or flex the neck slowly as the cup glides away from the neck and releases the soft tissue from the vacuum within the cup (figure 12.4).

Advanced Neck Cupping Techniques

There are three advanced techniques that I would like to demonstrate for the cervical spine. They take advantage of the deep soft-tissue manipulation created by the vacuum and the ability of this mechanism to deliver a firm stimulus that enhances movement and often reduces the sensitivity of the connective and contractile tissues around the neck. The techniques are specific and will not be suitable for all patients, especially those with high pain states.

Shearing

The neck shearing technique requires the vacuum to be maintained over the skin of the lower neck or upper shoulders without the cup sliding out of position. This then allows the combination of neck side flexion and cup manipulation in opposing directions

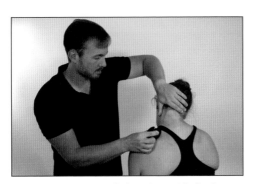

Figure 12.5. Cervical shearing with flexion and side flexion

to create the shearing force between the external pull of the cup and the internal pull from the neck (figure 12.5).

Vertebral Mobilization

The mobilization-with-movement technique uses the cup to create a vacuum around one of the lower cervical vertebrae by locating the cup centrally over C6, C7, or T1. The cup is then externally mobilized in accordance with the head rotation, so rotation of the head to the right would be aided by externally gliding the cup to the left to assist the rotation of the vertebrae (figure 12.6).

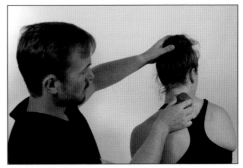

Figure 12.6. A single cup is used over C6, C7, or T1 to mobilize the neck through rotation

Mobilization

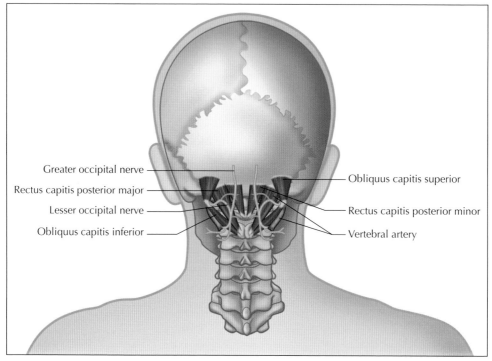

Greater occipital nerve

Rectus capitis posterior major

Lesser occipital nerve

Obliquus capitis inferior

Obliquus capitis superior

Rectus capitis posterior minor

Vertebral artery

Figure 12.7. The suboccipital muscles, vertebral artery, and suboccipital nerve

The Suboccipital Vacuum

The suboccipital muscles are a group of four muscles located between the top of the neck and the back of the head. They consist of four muscles, of which three form the borders of the suboccipital triangle, which surrounds the vertebral artery and suboccipital nerve on each side of the neck (figure 12.7). Manual therapy of the suboccipital region will often alleviate neck pain and tension and the associated headaches.

Cupping the suboccipital region can be difficult because hair often prevents the

creation of a vacuum. However, I always teach this technique on my courses and try it with my patients because when it does work, it is fantastically therapeutic and receives good feedback (figure 12.8).

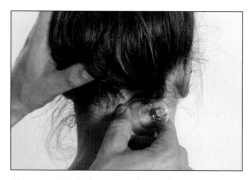

Figure 12.8. Suboccipital cupping

Conclusion

Cupping around the neck is one of my favorite strategies when working with neck-pain patients. There are so many ways to utilize the therapeutic benefits of a vacuum when treating neck pain that you will likely always find a method that suits your individual patient. I have found the active cupping techniques particularly useful for restoring neck function and reducing pain.

References

Chi, L.-M., L.-M. Lin, C.-L. Chen, S.-F. Wang, H.-L. Lai, and T.-C. Peng. 2016. The effectiveness of cupping therapy on relieving chronic neck and shoulder pain: A randomized controlled trial. *Evidence-Based Complementary and Alternative Medicine* 2016: 7358918.

Cohen, S.P. 2015. Epidemiology, diagnosis, and treatment of neck pain. *Mayo Clinic Proceedings* 90(2): 284–99.

Côté, P., J. D. Cassidy, and L. Carroll. 2003. The epidemiology of neck pain: What we have learned from our population-based studies. *Journal of the Canadian Chiropractic Association* 47(4): 284.

Hoy, D. G., M. Protani, R. De, and R. Buchbinder. 2010. The epidemiology of neck pain. *Best Practice and Research, Clinical Rheumatology* 24(6): 783–92.

Lauche, R., H. Cramer, C. Hohmann, K. E. Choi, T. Rampp, F. J. Saha, F. Musial, J. Langhorst, and G. Dobos. 2012. "The effect of traditional cupping on pain and mechanical thresholds in patients with chronic nonspecific neck pain: A randomised controlled pilot study." *Evidence-Based Complementary and Alternative Medicine* 2012: 429718.

Wirth, B., B. K. Humphreys, and C. Peterson. 2016. "Importance of psychological factors for the recovery from a first episode of acute non-specific neck pain: A longitudinal observational study." *Chiropractic and Manual Therapies* 24(1): 9.

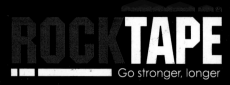
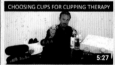 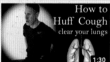
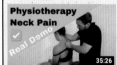 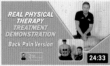 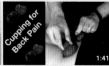 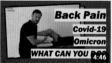 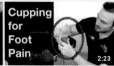 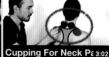